Alive Health

Recipe Book

Barbara J. Roberts

Author's Note: This book is intended as a reference only, not as specific medical advice.
The ideas, procedures, and suggestions contained herein are not intended to be a substitute
for consultation with your personal medical practitioner. The author shall not be liable or
responsible for any loss or damage allegedly arising from any information or suggestion in
this book. Further, if you suspect that you have a medical problem, I urge you to seek pro-
fessional medical help immediately.

Printed in the United States of America.   First Edition

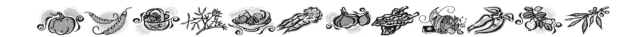

Table of Contents

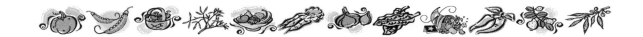

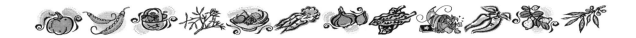

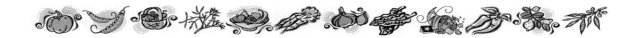

Main Meals 177

Crackers and Breads 189

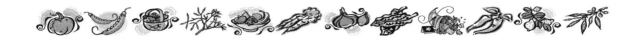

Desserts   205

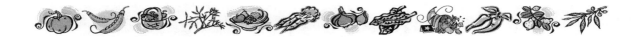

Beverages and Snacks

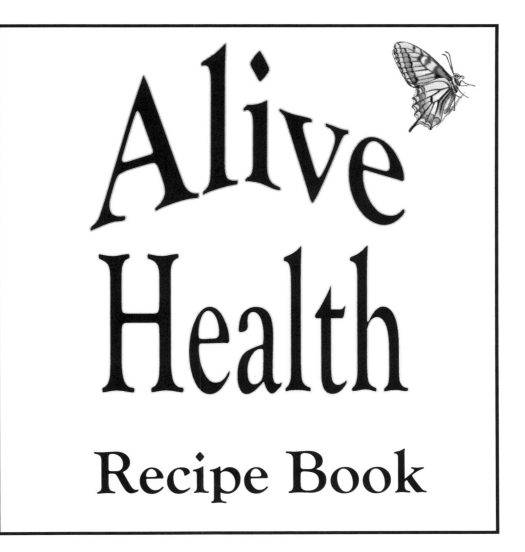

Alive Health

Recipe Book

PART ONE

Background Information

Preface

This book is the culmination of my passion to help people achieve optimal health through food and education. It offers quick and easy recipes for healthy eating on the run. This book also gives you the science behind what to avoid in your life and what to embrace.

Along the way, I hope to steer you around some of the pitfalls that I encountered when I started on this path in November of 2000. You can have healthy meals by spending just a portion of two days a week in the kitchen and then have enough good food to eat for an entire seven days.

To do this, you (or a willing recruit) must commit enough time to prepare the foods. You will also save money versus eating at fast food restaurants every day, even if you eat all organic. Best of all, your body will thank you for it.

About the recipes — one of my pet peeves is trying to read a recipe that goes from the bottom of one page to the top of another, so I made it a point to put each recipe on a single page. The book is printed in a large format so it will be easier to put into a book holder to use, and the recipes are printed in larger type to be easier on the eyes. (Those of us with older eyes know what a help that is!)

I would like to take this opportunity to thank my teachers in the raw food field, Brenda Cobb at the Living Foods Institute and Jackie and Gideon Graff at Sprout Raw Food. They encouraged and inspired me in my pursuit of better health, and in writing this book.

All of the baked goods made with coconut oil and flour were adapted from recipes by Dr. Bruce Fife, ND in his book "Cooking with Coconut Flour," Piccadilly books, Ltd. Other insight and stimulation came from Natalie Lussier from www.RawFoodsWitch.com.

Annette Mirsch assisted by expertly proof-reading the rough draft of my book and leaving valuable notes for me. Also, my neighbor, Paula R., was gracious enough to edit the manuscript, and for that I will be forever grateful.

I also want to thank Mary Ann Witcher and the members of the Georgia Farmgirls who were taste testers and opinion givers on several of my recipes. And last, but never least, I appreciate the patience, support, tasting and critiques of my dear partner in life, Brian Fraser, without whom I could not have done this.

I hope these recipes will inspire you to get in your kitchen and play. You can even get your kids involved in some of them. Who knows? They may learn to love kale – I know of one kid who does!

Here's to your health and happiness!

Introduction

What Constitutes Healthy Eating?

If you were to ask 50 different people what foods are healthy, you would get 50 different answers. To a certain extent, that's the way it should be, because there is no one-size-fits-all healthy eating plan that is right for everyone.

There are hundreds of ideas and opinions out there on how to eat healthy, and I am going to show you the one that has worked for me. My aim is to give you healthy substitutions for America's favorite foods.

My recipes are wheat-free, gluten-free, sugar-free, artificial sweetener-free, and most of all, guilt-free. They are mostly raw, except for the baked goods and meat. In addition, they actually taste good - I wouldn't be eating them if they weren't delicious!

I know, right now you are thinking, "Raw foods? Yuck!" and are summoning up images of "rabbit food." But there is much more to raw foods, and you will be amazed at the combinations you can come up with.

The main advantage of eating raw food is that it is simple and speedy. Raw food is easy to fix and transport. Plus, since it's a whole lot easier to keep something cold than hot, you can bypass the line at the office microwave!

In all things dealing with health, your body is the best gauge of what is right for you, no matter what anyone says. If you are tuned in to your body, it will give you clues as to what works for you and what doesn't. If something doesn't resonate with you, or work for you after sincerely trying it, then don't do it. The only expert on your health is YOU.

On the other hand, if something just seems different from what you are used to, or seems "weird," I urge you to go ahead and see if you might like it before automatically dismissing the idea. It could make a world of difference to you and your health.

How to tell if you are eating healthy foods

The system I follow was developed by Dr. Joseph Mercola. His wisdom on the subject of nutrition is the backbone of my beliefs. Dr. Mercola's nutritional typing has worked better for me than anything else I have ever tried and is presented in detail later in this book.

The plan has three distinct nutritional or body types — carbohydrate type, protein type or mixed type. Here's how to know if what you are eating is right for your particular type.

Generally speaking, eating right for your body type should make a lasting improvement in your energy, mental capacity, and emotional well-being. If, an hour or so after eating, you feel hungry even though you are physically full, crave sweets, your energy level drops, or you feel hyper, nervous, angry, irritable or depressed, then you are not eating the right foods for your body type.

For holistic health, you will need to become an expert label reader. By minimizing (or preferably eliminating) processed foods, you will not have to do it very much.

Things to look out for on labels are monosodium glutamate (MSG) or many of its aliases, trans fats (listed as either hydrogenated or partially hydrogenated vegetable oils), sugar, and anything ending in "ose", such as dextrose, maltose, sucralose, etc.

Avoid all of these. Later chapters in this book will give you more details on why to avoid them, plus list other things to look out for.

Buy locally or grow your own food

One of the easiest ways to be sure of what is in your food is to either buy locally from farmers that you know personally, or to grow the food yourself. Many local growers use organic methods, but are not certified because of the extra time and expense involved. You can also find out if a farmer is using any genetically modified crops (GMOs) if you contact them personally.

If you grow your own food, you have total control over what goes in the soil and on the plants. Therefore, you can have organic food easily. I'll give you some tips on organic gardening later.

This way of healthy eating will give your body the tools it needs to help keep you free of disease, and to aid in natural healing. When your body is in top notch condition, it can better ward off any harmful bacteria or viruses that come along.

In summary, your body will thank you for choosing this path for both yourself and your family. It will allow you to be in control of your health, with the cooperation of a compassionate health care provider who works in partnership with you.

A word about heating food: it is far better for your health if you do not ever use a microwave oven. The section on this will tell you why and give you alternative things that you can use to heat up necessities such as hot drinks, soups, popcorn, etc. That's another good reason to eat only raw foods - you don't have to heat them.

I do know that during the winter, your body craves hot foods so I have given you plenty of ways to have those. I don't want you to feel deprived in any way – there are so many great alternatives out there if you are willing to experiment!

Chapter 1

Why Eat Raw and Living Foods?

There has been much debate over the relative benefits of eating raw versus cooked food. I will give you a quick overview below. However, I personally eat raw foods because they're quicker and simpler to fix, and much easier to store and take with me as meals. There's no need to heat them up or try to keep them warm, and you can literally grab them out of the refrigerator and go. I like simplicity in my life.

So why eat raw and living foods? The heat from cooking destroys enzymes that our bodies need to digest food. Raw foods have all the enzymes that we need and they are still intact. Metabolic, digestive and food enzymes transform food into alkaline detoxifiers that neutralize the acid of our highly acidic cooked diet. Enzymes are critically necessary for achieving a balanced pH, as well as a balanced diet.

Acid/Alkaline balance

Our bodies, which should be more alkaline, are made acidic by virtue of the Standard American Diet (SAD). Cooked and processed foods are acidic. However, our organs prefer a neutral pH, and raw foods are alkaline, which puts our bodies back into equilibrium.

Heat destroys many vitamins, changing them so they cannot be fully absorbed by the body. Enzymes are also deactivated by heat, and by mechanical and chemical reactions. These are found not only in cooking, but also in the high temperatures involved in food processing and manufacturing, and the handling and storage of food. (This is addressed in the section on "Dirty Secrets of the Food Processing Industry," found on page 42)

If we eat a predominantly processed, synthesized, cooked, microwaved or convenience style diet, up to 90% of the enzymes and other vital nutrients are destroyed or rendered unavailable. So we end up as malnourished as the starving children in Africa, just at the other end of the spectrum.

White blood cells are triggered to increase when the body detects foreign substances. Cooking, refining, processing and adding chemicals to food alters the food to the point that the body does not recognize it, so white cells increase. This is called pathological leukocytosis.

The worst offenders are high heat processed foods, including beer, refined carbohydrates such as white flour and rice, and homogenized, pasteurized or preserved foods.

Raw plant foods are rich in oxygenating, alkalinizing chlorophyll. With live foods, the whole is greater than the sum of its parts in that the nutrients act synergistically with each other. Organic produce has an average of 83% more nutrients, as well.

Homeostasis

The body is always working towards homeostasis, or balance within its systems. We need a balance between raw and cooked foods, as well. If you can't eat your veggies raw, then at least steam them lightly or stir fry them for the best retention of nutrients. Eggs are best eaten raw, and meat should be cooked low and slow. I'll give you more specific information on eggs and meat in later sections.

Ideally, you should eat 85% of your food raw, and 15% of it cooked. Raw food is alive! Here is a fascinating article on the subject from Dr. Mercola's site: *http://articles.mercola.com/ sites/articles/archive/2009/03/21/Eat-Your-Food-Uncooked-Heres-the-Really-Raw-Truth.aspx*

Raw Foods Guidelines

A raw food diet is, in many ways, a lot easier to fix and eat than a cooked one. Foods travel much easier and you don't have to worry about heating things up. Why do you think sandwiches are so popular?

The best way to accomplish changing to a natural healing way of eating is to start slowly. Just try adding one new healthy dish at a time, substituting it for an established one, and go from there.

Hopefully, you can learn from my mistakes. I was so fired up after taking my first class that I made too many raw foods at once. Being organic, they went bad before I could eat them all. I didn't have any plan of action and threw out way too much stuff, a very expensive mistake.

That's one thing eating raw foods does require — planning ahead. After you get used to it, though, it's no big deal. Remember, if you fail to plan, you are planning to fail.

It's pretty much a given that around noon on most days, you are going to need to eat something. The same thing goes for mornings and evenings. So don't wait until those times to decide what you are going to eat. Plan in advance, and prepare accordingly. (This takes a lot of pressure off of you, too. Who hasn't come home from work and stressed out over what to fix for dinner?!)

A word of caution

If you jump into a totally raw foods diet without transitioning first, it may send you into *major* detox, so I advise against doing that. (You'll see why in a minute.) Gradually add in raw foods and monitor how you feel. Any amount of raw food that you can add to your daily diet will be beneficial to you.

Detoxing from eating raw foods may send you into what is called the Herxheimer reaction, sometimes called Herx or Herxing for short. It is also referred to as a Healing Crisis. In short, you'll feel worse before you feel better.

This is a very common effect and is to be embraced because it means that you are making a wonderful, vital difference in your life: you are cleaning out your system and gaining holistic health. Slowly transitioning into a raw foods diet will help minimize the symptoms of the Herxheimer reaction.

The Herxheimer Reaction

(from Jordan Rubin's newsletter)

"Is it ever good to feel bad? In some cases, yes. When you start a new treatment for an illness, your symptoms might increase at first, leaving you wondering if you're really getting healthier at all. This is called a Herxheimer reaction.

This is the "die-off" effect that many people experience when they dramatically improve their diet and lifestyles. It is an allergic response to the toxic by-products produced when the body's pH is changed for the better. When this happens, large numbers of dangerous bacteria and yeast organisms die and leave the body.

During this period, you won't feel very well, but in reality, you are responding positively to treatment. After this initial detoxification period, you should see significant improvement of your symptoms."

These symptoms may manifest themselves as making you feel as if you have the flu or a bad cold, but the mucous is just draining toxins from your body. Hang in there and see it through—it will be well worth it.

Beginning Guidelines

A few beginning guidelines for a raw food diet:

1. Try to buy organic foods whenever possible, even though the price is higher than for conventionally grown food. Our local grocery stores are doing a great job of providing these as often as possible, but you will have to go to a more organically-inclined market like Whole Foods or Natural Foods Warehouse to get some items.

2. Always soak raw raisins, dates, nuts and sun-dried tomatoes. The first two are soaked (for one to two hours) because they take fluid from the body if not pre-moistened. Nuts are soaked (for eight hours) to remove enzyme inhibitors, so always pour off the water from them. Don't use sun-dried tomatoes packed in oil, because of the preservatives. Instead, soak the dried tomatoes for at least two hours. This will prevent your food processor from bouncing all over the counter top when you try to process them.

3. Soak beans (like garbanzos) just until they have a little "tail" coming out of them. If you soak them too much and the tails are longer, they will taste bitter.

4. Use a Vitamix blender if possible, as they can take the severe use. All of the raw recipes will fit into a seven to eight-cup food processor, which is also a good item to have.

5. A rule of thumb for peeling raw fruits and vegetables: if they can sit out on your kitchen counter for a week and be okay, then they have enzyme inhibitors on them and must be peeled or carefully washed (apples, bananas, oranges, avocados, etc.). If they need to be refrigerated to keep (zucchini, squash, bell peppers etc.), they can be eaten as is. One exception is cucumbers, but that is because they are waxed.

6. Use only filtered, bottled or "good" well water at all times. This is very important if you want to have optimal health.

7. All measurements are the pre-soaked amounts, i.e. one cup of raw almonds or raisins *before* they are soaked. The volume will increase dramatically after soaking.

8. Lemon juice is our only preservative in raw foods and you will use it often. I personally do not buy organic lemons, unless I am going to use the zest of one, as they are pretty expensive. Just be sure to wash the conventional ones well with "Veggie Wash" or an eco-friendly soap such as "Seventh Generation."

9. To get pesticides off produce, you may want to investigate purchasing a Lotus Sanitizing System. This does work very well, but it is a bit pricey and isn't totally necessary. Otherwise wash items well, as instructed with the lemons.

10. Raw nuts are what we use to create "creaminess" in recipes such as salad dressings or "cheese" sauces. The most common ones used for this are macadamia nuts, pine nuts and brazil nuts. They need to be soaked before using. Purchase nuts from an organic market if possible. In a pinch, you can buy jarred or canned nuts, but they will be roasted and salted.

11. I use lots of coconut oil and extra virgin olive oil in my raw food recipes and these should both be organic. The coconut oil can be ordered by the gallon from Dr. Mercola's site (www.mercola.com/products), as well as purchased at some local grocery stores in smaller quantities.

12. When you use garlic, it should always be raw and as fresh as possible. Ideally, you should eat a few cloves of freshly crushed raw garlic a day, but I realize that it is not always possible to do this.

All cloves of garlic are not created equal. A normal clove of garlic should be about one inch in length and about a quarter inch in width. If you get a bigger one, count it as two or three in the recipes. Judge according to size. When peeling garlic, you can use the flat side of a knife to crush the clove first (improves flavor, too). Then the skin comes off easily.

If you make too much of a raw recipe and can't finish it all, it is okay to freeze it, although you lose about 20% of the nutrients by doing so. Still, this is preferable to throwing it out.

I take my food with me everywhere I go, even on trips. By putting it in individual containers, I can grab and go if necessary (as it often is). So, you can have fast food after all! I call it Grab and Go Goodness.

Grab and Go Goodness

Optimal health is a lot easier to achieve when the foods you eat are all literally Grab and Go. That's what I love most about them – they're quick to fix and take with me. (They have to be, with my crazy schedule!)

All of the recipes I included had to meet certain criteria before they could be added to the book or my website. They had to be wheat-free, gluten-free, sugar-free and artificial sweetener-free, as well as being fast and simple to fix. Many are even vegan.

I tried to make sure that you aren't left with ingredients you can't use in another recipe, because using organic ingredients means they don't store well for long periods.

Most of the recipes are raw, except for the baked goods that use coconut flour and coconut oil, both of which are extremely good for you.

Always take food with you

I was a massage therapist at a local resort in the North Georgia mountains and I didn't know from one day to the next whether I would have any massages scheduled. So, I may have planned a day to do errands and the night before find out that I have two massages to do. Or I might go to the Spa thinking I have two massages to do and end up with six.

To have healthy food with me at all times, I carried my lunch with me wherever I went. It was too far from work to go back home to eat, and I may not have had time, anyway. Plus, there are absolutely no food places closer than 15 minutes away from the resort.

Because I am blessed to live across the valley from Amicalola Falls, one of Georgia's most beautiful state parks, I have to travel 20 minutes to get to a bank, post office, grocery store or any kind of "civilization." It's 30 minutes to GA Highway 400 where my favorite grocery store, Kroger, is located.

When I go out to do errands, it may take the whole day because I save them up to do all at once. So again, I always take my lunch with me to ensure healthy eating for my body.

How do I do it?

Every recipe I make has enough to last at least four days for one person. If you have a family to feed, adjust accordingly.

When I make a large recipe, I put it into smaller containers such as food-grade plastic ones with lids. I know that it would be better to use glass, as it is more inert and won't leach anything out, but I have to be practical. Glass breaks too easily and won't fit into my cooler with most of the lids which are designed for the containers.

I use left-over tubs from things like miso or peanut butter (from make your own places). These are usually 16-ounce sizes and I fill them to the top. That way I am getting four servings of vegetables for optimal health and I don't have to take anything else with me.

Whole Foods carries packages of Applegate Farms chicken and turkey meat. One package is several birds put together in a single parcel. These are organic and pre-cooked with only salt, water and paprika as seasonings, so they are ready to use and there is no waste.

I buy the chicken or turkey, cut it up into three-ounce portions, and freeze them in two-serving packages. Since a three-ounce portion is the size of a deck of cards, I frequently get a deck out to make sure I haven't over-estimated as I cut them up.

Each day, I take out what I need and put it into the refrigerator to thaw. As soon as I finish one package, I take another one out of the freezer to have it ready for the next two days.

You can alternatively cook up four pieces of pork chops or a steak and use that instead. I normally use boneless because that way I can eat them more easily with one hand while I'm driving. (Yes, I know I shouldn't, but I do.) Also, I don't have to worry about bones and having them smell and attract critters. Since we do have bears up here, that is a real problem. However, if cost is a factor, by all means buy bone-in cuts.

How to carry your lunch with you

Use a small cooler or insulated bag to actually carry your lunch with you as you go about your daily routine. I use a plain, six-pack Coleman-type cooler that you can pick up anywhere during hot weather. Buy some of those small blue ice packs (mine are Rubbermaid brand) that fit in easily.

I take one of the small blue ice packs and put it in one corner of my six-pack Coleman cooler. To eat, I use old mismatched cutlery instead of plastic, since metal is safer to use. If you go to my website and look under "Raw Living Recipes – Grab and Go Goodness" (from the Site Map), you can see pictures of all of these.

Then I put the meat in its packaging on top of the ice pack. The veggie container goes to the side of the it, with a dessert of some kind (muffins, GORP bars, etc.) on top.

If you use the healthy chocolate recipe, be sure to put it on the blue ice pack too since it will melt at 76 ° F. It will definitely melt in your hand, not in your mouth, if it is summertime!

And there you have it – healthy eating on the run! I just change out the meat and veggies each day and have a small variety of healthy desserts to take along with me to satisfy my sweet tooth.

For dinner when I get home, I choose a veggie container again, and a meat (usually one I cook such as grass-finished ground beef or Coleman brand chicken sausages). If I feel particularly fancy that evening, I put them on a plate. If not, I eat them out of the containers (frequently in front of the computer, which I know is not optimal) and that gives me one less thing to wash.

I choose to eat to live, rather than living to eat, and the health benefits for me have been enormous. Rarely do I depart from this routine and I don't have cravings. I also don't eat as much as I used to. I'm simply not hungry and the amounts I do eat satisfy me very well.

Traveling for several days with your own food

In a former life, I used to videotape Ballroom Dance competitions around the country. I also taught dancing for 26 years. To avoid having to eat hotel food or fast food, I would take my own food with me.

To do this, I first tried taking a large rolling cooler with me with ice packs from home. But at a hotel, I would have to put ice in to try to keep things cold and then would have a problem with it melting and leaking out. Plus, it did not keep items cold enough and I ended up getting sick one time from spoiled food.

But then I discovered this great cooler from Coleman that has a plug which goes into a car cigarette lighter (see pictures on the same page on my website) and keeps food cold that way. You can also turn the cord around and heat up things in it. No more spoiled food, and the cooler kept it at a good temperature!

The cooler has an electric adapter that allows you to plug it in when you get to your destination. That worked perfectly for me. I just put it on a rolling stand to take through airports and had healthy food whenever I wanted it, even on the plane. Check your clothing luggage and carry the food on with you if you are really serious about optimal health.

Of course, with the new TSA rules for flying, you would need to check with the airport where you are originating for the rules and regulations that apply these days. It may be that they won't allow this type of thing anymore. I have heard horror stories about it.

Nutritional Typing

For optimum health, the best system I have tried is Dr. Mercola's nutritional typing. He tried, as did I, for many years to find a viable and doable eating plan.

Dr. Mercola had the resources to research what works and what doesn't through his clinic outside of Chicago and this is what he finally decided was the best system. It has worked very well for me, and has given me the energy and stamina that I desired.

Here is an overview of the plan. The best thing to do, though, is to go to his website and take the test to see which type you are. The test can be found on his site and is currently free for a limited time only: http://products.mercola.com/nutritional-typing.

The different nutritional types

I briefly mentioned the three nutritional types earlier. Here they are in more detail as I promised you.

Protein types should eat high protein of certain kinds, with a restricted carbohydrate and relatively high fat (healthy fats only) emphasis.

Carbo types should eat mostly carbohydrates, but be selective about which ones. (There is a major difference between vegetables and grains.) They should eat some specific kinds of meat also, for optimum health.

Mixed types should eat some protein, carbohydrates, and healthy fats. This type is the most challenging of all because it takes really listening to your body to determine what foods are optimal for you.

The order in which you eat your food is important. Protein types should eat protein first and carbo types should eat their carbohydrates first. Mixed types should eat both together. The commonly touted "eat a variety of foods at each meal" is really best for mixed types.

I happen to be a mixed type, and while I am grateful for the variety of foods that I can have, it has been difficult to find out exactly which foods are best for me. Determining that involves *really listening* to your body and how it reacts to everything you eat, and everything you *put on* your body, as well.

For a quick and VERY oversimplified way to tell which type you are, gauge your reaction to red meat and orange juice. If you can't abide the idea of eating red meat (physically, not just ideologically), then you are most likely a carbo type.

If you cannot stomach orange juice, you are most likely a protein type. If you like both, then you are a mixed type. One other option would be to purchase Dr. Mercola's book, "Take Control of Your Health," which outlines it pretty well.

What you will receive when you sign up on Dr. Mercola's site:

You will get a chart of what foods are best for your type, plus relevant tips for your particular type and information on nutrition in general.

Once you understand the principles behind a diet based on nutritional typing, it is pretty easy to follow. I highly recommend taking the test, as it will tell you a great deal.

There is great information here for the best healthy eating you can find. As always, though, if anything doesn't resonate with you, you should not do it. Everyone has a unique makeup.

Chapter 2

What To Avoid

As mentioned in the introduction, the foods you should avoid are wheat, gluten, sugar, and artificial sweeteners. We will look at each of these individually, and explain why they should not be part of your diet.

Grains

The grains that most of America eats should ideally be avoided for a number of reasons. Primarily, most grains, even organic whole grains, turn into sugar in the human body almost immediately. This in turn perpetuates the progression towards diabetes and obesity, which are becoming epidemic in today's society.

Here is a quote on this subject taken from Dr. Mercola's excellent health education website: "Grains and sugars are often an overlooked addiction and the way to manage any addiction is though complete abstinence.

The reason most people struggle with giving up sugar is that they are still eating grains. The grains break down to sugar and perpetuate the addiction. Eliminating grains and sugars and eating properly for your nutritional type are the keys to optimal health." *(http:// articles.mercola.com/sites/articles/archive/2004/12/04/grains.aspx)*

Problems with wheat

Wheat is especially problematic. It is considered to be the staff of life and yet it causes more problems than other grains, likely because of its pervasiveness in American society today.

If wheat were still harvested as it was hundreds of years ago, it would have greater nutritional value. In the old days, when wheat was harvested, it was left in the fields for a few days and it partially sprouted from the dew. That enhanced its nutrition greatly.

Wheat was also ground using stones, which left most of the beneficial bran still intact. This is what was so nutritious. (Remember in *Heidi,* where she kept the nutritionally deficient white rolls to take back to her Alm Uncle, thinking they were so much better?)

There is an article by Jen Allbritton entitled "Wheaty indiscretions: What Happens to Wheat from Seed to Storage," that gives more insight into what really happens with modern day farming. The full article can be found here: *(http://articles.mercola.com/sites/articles/archive/2003/07/26/avoid-wheat.aspx)*

Gluten intolerance

Many people today are gluten sensitive, if not downright intolerant of it. This is referred to as celiac disease. It is estimated to affect as many as 1 out of 10 Americans, but the number could actually be much higher.

Because it turns into glucose in the body, over-consumption of grains often leads to insulin resistance. Insulin resistance is a pre-cursor to diabetes and all of the problems that come with it. Some of the symptoms include:

- Fatigue
- Brain fog
- Low blood sugar (or hypoglycemia)
- Intestinal bloating
- Sleepiness
- Increased fat storage and weight gain
- Increased triglycerides
- Increased blood pressure
- Depression

Here's an explanation of gluten intolerance from Dr. Mercola's informative website:

"In a nutshell, even though carbohydrates themselves are fat-free, excess carbohydrates end up as excess fat. That's not the worst of it. Any meal or snack high in carbohydrates will generate a rapid rise in blood glucose. To adjust for this rapid rise, the pancreas secretes the hormone insulin into the bloodstream. Insulin then lowers the levels of blood glucose.

The problem is that insulin is essentially a storage hormone, evolved to put aside excess carbohydrate calories in the form of fat in case of future famine. So the insulin that's stimulated by excess carbohydrates aggressively promotes the accumulation of body fat. In other words, when we eat too much carbohydrate, we're essentially sending a hormonal message, via insulin, to the body (actually, to the adipose cells). The message: "Store fat."
(www.mercola.com/article/carbohydrates/lower_your_grains.htm)

Soaking grains

One other aspect of grains is that, if you are going to eat them, you need to soak them first to remove antinutrients from them. This info is from Sally Fallon:

"Grains require careful preparation because they contain a number of antinutrients that can cause serious health problems. Phytic acid, for example, is an organic acid in which phosphorus is bound. It is mostly found in the bran or outer hull of seeds. Untreated phytic acid can combine with calcium, magnesium, copper, iron and especially zinc in the intestinal tract and block their absorption."

"Other antinutrients in whole grains include enzyme inhibitors which can inhibit digestion and put stress on the pancreas; irritating tannins; complex sugars which the body cannot break down; and gluten and related hard-to-digest proteins which may cause allergies, digestive disorders and even mental illness.

Proper preparation of grains is a kind and gentle process that imitates the process that occurs in nature. It involves soaking for a period in warm, acidulated water in the preparation of porridge, or long, slow sour dough fermentation in the making of bread. Such processes neutralize phytic acid and enzyme inhibitors."

Changes in the way wheat is grown

Sally continues on the subject:

"Bread can be the staff of life, but modern technology has turned our bread—even our whole grain bread—into a poison. Grains are laced with pesticides during the growing season and in storage; they are milled at high temperatures so that their fatty acids turn rancid. Rancidity increases when milled flours are stored for long periods of time, particularly in open bins.

The bran and germ are often removed and sold separately, when Mother Nature intended that they be eaten together with the carbohydrate portion; they're baked as quick rise breads so that antinutrients remain; synthetic vitamins and an unabsorbable form of iron added to white flour can cause numerous imbalances; dough conditioners, stabilizers, preservatives and other additives add insult to injury.

Cruelty to grains in the making of breakfast cereals is intense. Slurries of grain are forced through tiny holes at high temperatures and pressures in giant extruders, a process that destroys nutrients and turns the proteins in grains into veritable poisons. Westerners pay a lot for expensive breakfast cereals that snap, crackle and pop, including the rising toll of poor health.

The final indignity to grains is that we treat them as loners, largely ignorant of other dietary factors needed for the nutrients they provide. Fat-soluble vitamins A and D found in animal fats like butter, lard and cream help us absorb calcium, phosphorus, iron, B vitamins and the many other vitamins that grains provide. Porridge eaten with cream will do us a thousand times more good than cold breakfast cereal with skim milk; sourdough whole grain bread with butter or whole cheese is a combination that contributes to optimal health.

Be kind to your grains. . . and your grains will deliver their promise as the staff of life. Buy only organic whole grains and soak them overnight to make porridge or casseroles; or grind them into flour with a home grinder and make your own sour dough bread and baked goods. For those who lack the time for breadmaking, kindly-made whole grain breads are now available. Look for organic, stone ground, sprouted or sour dough whole grain breads and enjoy them with butter or cheese." *(This article can be found on the Weston A. Price website at www.westonaprice.org under "Be Kind To Your Grains.")*

Other problems with wheat

Another problem with commercially made wheat products today is that they often contain Potassium Bromate as dough extenders. "When you ingest or absorb bromine, it displaces iodine, and this iodine deficiency leads to an increased risk for cancer of the breast, thyroid gland, ovary and prostate -- cancers that we see at alarmingly high rates today." *(http://blogs. mercola.com/sites/vitalvotes/archive/2009/07/09/another-poison-hiding-in-your-environment.aspx)*

The final reason for avoiding grain products is that American wheat is bred to have a higher gluten content compared to European wheat. This increases the potential for gluten sensitivity. According to Dr. Mercola, "Gluten is the primary protein found in wheat. In my experience, there is an epidemic of hidden intolerance to wheat products. There are frequently no obvious symptoms.

Rice, corn, buckwheat and millet have glutens, but the glutens in these foods do not contain the gliadin molecule that can provoke the inflammatory reaction. Therefore, they are usually safe. Other safe grains include quinoa and amaranth.

Gliadins are molecules that frequently cause toxic reactions that trigger your immune response. ...This immune response damages surrounding tissue and has the potential to set off, or exacerbate, MANY other health problems throughout your body, which is why gluten can have such a devastating effect on your overall health." *(http://www.mercola.com/nutritionplan/beginner.htm)*

The most common symptoms of gluten intolerance are abdominal pain, diarrhea and fatigue, which can be caused by any number of different things. My personal experience was an almost constant abdominal cramping, gas, bloating, diarrhea and weight gain.

I thought that it was normal to feel that way, and only by eliminating grains did I find out that it was not. If I only do it occasionally, I can still have some wheat, but I usually pay for it with ill health the next day.

If you take the steps to eliminate all harmful grains from your diet, you will see an amazing change in your overall health. Just eliminate the major offenders and see how you feel.

Then, for optimal health, try the gluten-free recipes on this site and compare your daily health afterwards. Healthy eating can also utilize good-tasting food. You just have to be willing to experiment and try new things.

Sugar

For an in-depth look at exactly how sugar is harmful, please watch the video called "Sugar: The Bitter Truth" that can be found on Dr. Mercola's site, along with a pretty disgusting "ad" for high fructose corn syrup (HFCS). Here is the address*: http://articles.mercola.com/sites/articles/archive/2010/01/02/HighFructose-Corn-Syrup-Alters-Human-Metabolism.aspx*

The video will make you think twice before eating sugar ever again and should be required viewing for all of the American people. It tells us that in the last 20 years, we have increased sugar consumption in the U.S. to 135 lbs. of sugar per person per year! Prior to the turn of this century (1887-1890), the average consumption was only 5 lbs. per person per year.

One other reason to do away with sugar is that the FDA just recently approved genetically modified sugar beets. So unless you like eating "Frankenfoods," your best bet is to buy organic sugar if you must have it, or at least make sure you are getting cane sugar, instead of sugar from beets.

I buy cane sugar for my hummingbird feeders because they're my favorite birds and I don't want to take a chance on hurting them in any way. That way I know it's safe.

Benefits of no longer eating sugar

Eliminating sugar was extremely difficult for me at first, until I addressed so many of the other issues I was facing. It definitely was affecting my adrenal glands, which were already suffering from too much abuse. I was finally able to eliminate Candida from my body, which I thought would never happen.

I no longer have hypoglycemia and, as long as I stick to the principles of my nutritional type (Mixed Type), I can go for six or more hours without eating, and I don't feel hungry. My energy level is up, I don't feel "brain fog" anymore, and all of my numbers are where they should be for triglycerides, cholesterol, and fasting blood sugar.

I no longer have cravings for sweets (that took a LONG time) and processed baked goods hold no appeal to me at all. Only a chocolate chip cookie can occasionally call to me – that's the one thing I might succumb to eating.

In short, I am on my way to optimal health now and have a new healthy way of eating, with grab and go goodness. You can, too, by following the principles set out in this book.

Artificial Sweeteners

Some of the most dangerous substances to come on the market lately, in my opinion, are all the artificial sweeteners. Unfortunately, Americans are so addicted to sugar that some form of sweetener is mandatory in the Standard American Diet (SAD) today.

Most of the artificial sweeteners on the market now should not be consumed for a multitude of reasons. If Mother Nature didn't make it, you should not be eating it. Products made in a lab are bound to cause problems sooner or later because your body does not recognize these things.

Dr. Joseph Mercola is one of the leading authorities on this subject and has actually written a book on it titled *Sweet Deception*. This excellent book will give you all of the facts and figures as to how these products were developed and how they got approved and put out in the marketplace.

I'm going to cover just a few of these and let you visit his web site for articles on the other kinds of fake sweeteners. All of them are to be avoided, and happily, there are plenty of great substitutes. I'm going to provide you with a few quotes from some of Dr. Mercola's articles to give you a sampling.

Aspartame

Aspartame, under brand names NutraSweet® and Equal®, is the worst offender, according to Dr. Mercola in this article: *http://articles.mercola.com/sites/articles/archive/2009/ 10/13/Artificial-Sweeteners-More-Dangerous-than-You-Ever-Imagined.aspx.* It offers a wealth of information concerning this danger and I highly advise reading it. It gives you symptoms to check for and resources for what to do to eliminate them.

According to the article, the FDA has more reports of adverse side effects from this sweetener than any other product. Among these are: headache, change in mood, change in vision, convulsions and seizures, sleep problems/insomnia, change in heart rate, hallucination, abdominal cramps/pain, memory loss, rash, nausea and vomiting, fatigue and weakness, dizziness/poor equilibrium, diarrhea, hives, and joint pain.

Aspartame is a neurological excitotoxin that can cause extensive damage. "The term *excitotoxicity* was coined by Dr. Russell Blaylock, a neurosurgeon[12]. It describes the ability of certain amino acids like monosodium glutamate (MSG) and aspartic acid to literally excite cells to death." This particularly applies to brain cells.

This artificial sweetener can also lead to weight *gain.* Yes, what you are ingesting to help you control your weight is actually doing just the opposite. To quote again from the article: "The two main ingredients of aspartame, phenylalanine and aspartic acid, stimulate the release of insulin and leptin -- hormones which instruct your body to store fat.

In addition, a large intake of phenylalanine can drive down your serotonin levels. Serotonin is the neurotransmitter that tells you when you're full. A low level of serotonin can bring on food cravings which can lead to weight gain.[20]"

Neotame™ is the "new and improved version" but is likely to be just as detrimental to your health as aspartame. *Parents, be aware that aspartame is frequently found in children's vitamins, especially the name brands like Flintstones. Be particularly alert to this danger.*

Splenda™ (Sucralose)

McNeil Nutritionals, the makers of Splenda, would have you believe that it is "made from sugar so it tastes like sugar." Yes, it's sugar, but with a few chlorine molecules added which makes it not like sugar at all! The sugar industry is currently suing McNeil Nutritionals for implying that Splenda is a natural form of sugar with no calories.

From this excellent in-depth article on Splenda found on Dr. Mercola's website I quote: "In the five step patented process of making sucralose, three chlorine molecules are added to a sucrose or sugar molecule. A sucrose molecule is a disaccharide that contains two single sugars bound together; glucose and fructose.

The chemical process to make sucralose alters the chemical composition of the sugar so much that it is somehow converted to a fructo-galactose molecule. This type of sugar molecule does not occur in nature and therefore your body does not possess the ability to properly metabolize it. As a result of this "unique" biochemical make-up, McNeil Nutritionals makes its claim that Splenda is not digested or metabolized by the body, making it have zero calories. ...If your body had the capacity to metabolize it then it would no longer have zero calories."

As to how much Splenda is absorbed into your body, it varies with the individual. "Some of you will absorb and metabolize more than others. If you are healthy and your digestive system works well, you may be at higher risk for breaking down this product in your stomach and intestines. Please understand that it is impossible for the manufacturers of Splenda to make any guarantees based on their limited animal data."

"The entire issue of long-term safety has never been established. Let's look at the facts again: There have only been six human trials to date, the longest trial lasted three months, and at LEAST 15% of Splenda is not excreted from your body in a timely manner

Considering that Splenda bears more chemical similarity to DDT than it does to sugar, are you willing to bet your health on this data? Remember that fat soluble substances, such as DDT, can remain in your fat for decades and devastate your health." *(http:// articles.mercola.com/ sites/ articles/ archive/ 2000/ 12/ 03/ sucralose-dangers.aspx)*

Drinking water implications

Artificial sweeteners are found in drinking water now, along with all kinds of drug residues like statins, anti-depressants, blood thinners, etc., as people excrete them out of their bodies. Dr. Mercola explains:

"Sewage treatment plants fail to remove artificial sweeteners completely from waste water. These pollutants contaminate waters downstream, and may still be present in your drinking water.

A new, robust analytical method, which simultaneously extracts and analyzes seven commonly used artificial sweeteners, demonstrated the presence of several artificial sweeteners in waste water.

Until now, only sucralose has been detected in aquatic environments. Through the use of the new method, researchers were able to show for the first time that four artificial sweeteners -- acesulfame, saccharin, cyclamate, and sucralose -- are present in the waters from sewage treatment plants, indicating incomplete elimination during waste water treatment." *(http://blogs.mercola.com/sites/vitalvotes/archive/2009/06/19/the-bitter-side-of-artificial-sweeteners.aspx)*

Sugar Alcohols

One other class of sweeteners is the sugar alcohols. Dr. Mercola has this to say about them: "Sugar alcohols (also known as polyols) like erythritol are regulated as either GRAS (Generally Regarded As Safe) or food additives. Despite the name, sugar alcohols are neither sugar nor alcohol. They vary in sweetness from about half as sweet as sugar to equally as sweet.

They're frequently combined with other low-calorie or artificial sweeteners such as aspartame, acesulfame-K, neotame, saccharin, or as in the case of VitaminWater, crystalline fructose. The reason sugar alcohols provide fewer calories than sugar is because they are not completely absorbed in your body. However, this fact has certain drawbacks, none of which are good.

High intakes of foods containing sugar alcohols can lead to adverse physical symptoms like abdominal gas and diarrhea. Some polyols are clearly worse than others. Sorbitol or mannitol-containing foods, for example, are so potent they must display a warning on their label stating "excess consumption may have a laxative effect."

In connection with crystalline fructose, Dr. Mercola states that "While many people mistakenly believe that fructose is an acceptable form of sweetener, it is far from healthy. Refined man-made fructose metabolizes to triglycerides and adipose tissue, not blood glucose.

...Based on the latest research, crystalline fructose is definitely something you'll want to avoid as much as possible. Whereas regular HFCS contains 55 percent fructose and 45 percent glucose, crystalline fructose is at minimum *99 percent fructose*, which could only mean that all the health problems associated with fructose may be even more pronounced with this product. And if that's not bad enough, crystalline fructose may also contain arsenic, lead, chloride and heavy metals." *(http://articles.mercola.com/sites/articles/archive/2009/05/26/what-is-erythritol-doing-in-vitamin-water.aspx)*

The bottom line is that it is far safer to just totally eliminate all of the artificial sweeteners listed above. When you have reached optimum health, then you can *occasionally* indulge in the sugar only types of sweeteners.

Pure Via™ and Truvia®

Two other new sweeteners on the market are Pure Via and Truvia, which are made from the herb Stevia. While this is better, in that Stevia is a natural substance, for the makers to be able to patent it, it had to be artificially manipulated. My advice would be to stick to pure Stevia, which I am going to tell you about later on.

Fear not, I am going to give you some healthy alternatives to these evils so that you can still have some sweetness in your life with no guilt and no adverse side effects. After all, life is to be enjoyed!

MSG (Monosodium Glutamate)

The dangers of MSG

Most people think of MSG as an additive in Chinese food only, but that is not the case. MSG is in virtually every processed food on grocery shelves, from soups and crackers to meats and chips. It's also in most restaurants (especially fast food ones), and in school cafeterias, because it makes food taste good and is incredibly cheap, just like sugar.

According to Dr. Russell Blaylock, a board certified neurosurgeon and author of the highly recommended book *Excitotoxins: The Taste that Kills*, MSG is an excitotoxin (like Aspartame) which means that it overexcites your cells to the point of death and thus acts as a poison. It is also most likely a factor in the rising obesity epidemic we have in this country. When you ingest foods that contain MSG, your body produces visceral fat, the most dangerous kind. Visceral fat surrounds your internal body organs. It increases your risk of heart attack, stroke, type 2 diabetes and insomnia, just to name a few.

Avoiding MSG is difficult to do because it goes under so many different names. Therefore it is wisest to eat only natural, unprocessed food with ingredients that you can pronounce. Be on the look-out for these other names for MSG (from the literature), and ingredients high in glutamate.

"Natural flavorings" (very common and very deceptive)
2-aminoglutaric acid
Accent (remember "Wake up that flavor!"?)
Ajinomoto
Autolyzed yeast extract
Flavor enhancer 621
Gelatin

Hydrolyzed yeast
Malted Barley
Marmite
Rice Syrup or Brown Rice Syrup
Sodium glutamate
Soy extract
Soy sauce
Vegemite
Vetsin
Yeast Extract

Dr. Mercola has this to say about MSG: "Based on peer reviewed studies, there is no question that MSG is neurotoxic. It can cause blindness and many other problems such as headaches, fatigue, disorientation and depression." *http://articles.mercola.com/sites/articles/archive/2007/07/10/why-you-do-not-want-to-eat-processed-foods.aspx*

You won't hear about these dangers in the mainstream media because the food industry is too entrenched in using this poison. MSG retains the flavors of goods that have been sitting on a shelf for a long time and therefore acts as a preservative.

Since it is a flavor enhancer, it is found in all commercially prepared gravies, salad dressings and soups, especially diet ones. To make them diet, they take out the fat which leaves them bland tasting, and to make up for that, they put in MSG or one of its derivatives. Most of Campbell's soups contain them. It suppresses the immune system too, and what is the most common recommendation when you have a cold? Of course! Eat chicken soup, most likely from a can.

Diet foods and drinks contain MSG in some form to improve their flavor. Liquid amino acid preparations, such as soy sauce, have it as well.

Please be an informed consumer

These are serious issues that need to be addressed and I strongly urge you to become informed on this subject. Those who have tried to get this information out have been brutally suppressed, in many cases, and I commend Dr. Blaylock for his well-researched and documented references in his book and videos.

Dr. Mercola's article (referenced above) has more information about the dangers of MSG. I also strongly advise watching the hour long video about MSG from Dr. Russell Blaylock that can be found on the web site.

Genetically Modified Organisms (GMOs)

GMOs are one of the scariest things to come out of the 20th century, in my opinion. The worst thing is that we can't know what is genetically engineered (GE — another way of saying it) and what isn't. The only way to be sure is to buy organic, which, by law, cannot have any GE parts.

A video with Jeffrey Smith from Dr. Mercola's website *http://blogs.mercola.com/sites/ vitalvotes/archive/2009/09/29/everything-you-have-to-know-about-dangerous-genetically-modified- foods.aspx* gives you in-depth information about how GMOs are created. The FDA has been bought out as far as approval of these items is concerned.

Unless you are eating only organic foods that you have purchased or grown yourself, then you ARE eating GMOs. The worst thing is that the FDA, in its infinite wisdom, decreed that companies did not have to label these ingredients as such. So unless you make it your-self from organic ingredients, it most likely has genetically modified foods in it.

The following quote is also from Dr. Mercola: "Genetically modified crops are the result of a technology developed in the 1970s that allows genes from one species to be forced into the DNA of unrelated species. The inserted genes produce proteins that confer traits in the new plant, such as herbicide tolerance or pesticide production.

The process of creating the GM crop can produce all sorts of side effects. The plants con-tain proteins that have never existed before in the food supply.

In the US, new types of food substances are normally classified as food additives, which must undergo extensive testing, including long-term animal feeding studies.4 If approved, the label of food products containing the additive must list it as an ingredient.

Exceptions made for GRAS substances

An exception is made for substances that are deemed "generally recognized as safe" (GRAS). GRAS status allows a product to be commercialized without any additional testing.

Per US law, the substance must be the subject of a substantial amount of peer-reviewed published studies (or equivalent) to be considered GRAS. There must also be overwhelm-ing consensus among the scientific community that the product is safe.

GM foods met neither requirement. Nonetheless, in a precedent-setting move that some experts contend was illegal, the FDA declared in 1992 that GM crops are GRAS as long as their producers say they are. So the FDA does not require any safety evaluations or labels. A company can even introduce a GM food to the market without telling the agency. Such a lenient approach to GM crops was largely the result of Monsanto's legendary influence over the US government.

According to the New York Times, 'What Monsanto wished for from Washington, Monsanto and, by extension, the biotechnology industry, got... When the company abruptly decided that it needed to throw off the regulations and speed its foods to market, the White House quickly ushered through an unusually generous policy of self-policing.'" *(http://articles.mercola.com/sites/articles/archive/2007/10/23/what-else-do-biotech-companies-engineer.aspx)*

For a complete and thorough understanding of all of the implications of GE food, I suggest that you read the rest of the above referenced article in its entirety, or watch the Jeffrey Smith video. An in-depth review of GMOs can be found at *www.raw.wisdom.com/50harmful*.

For a list of genetically modified processed foods in categories that can be printed out, please go to this web site: *www.truefoodnow.org/shoppersguide/guide_printable.html*. It is an all-encompassing list and you can take this with you when you go shopping in the future. Your health, and the health of your loved ones, is at stake.

High Fructose Corn Syrup (HFCS)

High fructose corn syrup is one of the most insidious substances around in America today. It is estimated that fully one-quarter of the calories consumed by adolescents today comes from sodas, fruit juices, or pre-sweetened drinks, most of which contain HFCS.

Most people don't count those calories in their daily food intake, because they are hydration. Drinks aren't as filling as food is, so they take in far more calories than they realize.

This information from Dr. Mercola's website explains more about it. "It isn't that fructose itself is bad -- it is the MASSIVE DOSES you're exposed to that make it dangerous.

There are two reasons fructose is so damaging:

1. Your body metabolizes fructose in a much different way than glucose. The entire burden of metabolizing fructose falls on your liver.

2. People are consuming fructose in enormous quantities, which has made the negative effects much more profound.

Today, 55 percent of sweeteners used in food and beverage manufacturing are made from corn, and the number one source of calories in America is soda, in the form of HFCS. Food and beverage manufacturers began switching their sweeteners from sucrose (table sugar) to corn syrup in the 1970s when they discovered that HFCS was not only far cheaper to make, it's also about 20 times sweeter than table sugar.

This switch drastically altered the average American diet. By USDA estimates, about one-quarter of the calories consumed by the average American is in the form of added sugars, and most of that is HFCS. ...Making matters worse, all of the fiber has been removed from these processed foods, so there is essentially no nutritive value at all."

The differences in how sugars are metabolized

The article goes on to say that "After eating fructose, 100 percent of the metabolic burden rests on your liver. But with glucose, your liver has to break down only 20 percent.

Every cell in your body, including your brain, utilizes glucose. Therefore, much of it is "burned up" immediately after you consume it. By contrast, fructose ...get[s] stored as fat. ...Consuming fructose is essentially consuming fat!"

"Glucose suppresses the hunger hormone ghrelin and stimulates leptin, which suppresses your appetite. Fructose has no effect on ghrelin and interferes with your brain's communication with leptin, resulting in overeating.

The bottom line is: fructose leads to increased belly fat, insulin resistance and metabolic syndrome -- not to mention the long list of chronic diseases that directly result." *(http:// articles.mercola.com/ sites/ articles/ archive/ 2010/ 01/ 02/ HighFructose-Corn-Syrup-Alters-Human-Metabolism.aspx)*

So don't let anyone tell you now that High Fructose Corn Syrup is the same as sugar. And beware, they are changing the name of it too, to High Maltose Corn Syrup to deceive you even further.

HFCS is everywhere

In response to the growing body of scientific studies showing the dangers of HFCS, the Corn Refiner's Association launched a series of ads saying that it was fine to have HFCS "in moderation." Even if you choose to believe them, how in the world do you get it "in moderation"? It is everywhere!

If you eat processed foods of any kind, you are going to *have* to start reading labels. It is in almost all drinks (soda, pre-sweetened, energy, or fruit ones), candy, cookies, cakes, (almost all baked goods), some dairy products (yogurt), canned fruits and vegetables, ice cream, jams, jellies and syrups, some meats (especially Lunchables brand), sauces, soups, crackers, breads, cereals and worst of all in my opinion, *cough medicine*.

If you eat out in any restaurant, from fast food to high end, you are going to be eating GMOs, HFCS, or pesticide-laden food. Why? Because they are cheaper. Restaurants have to do this in order to make a profit.

Grocery stores are a little better, in that they give you a choice, but most of their products have the above items, especially processed foods. That's why you have to prepare your own food at home if you want optimum health.

Soy Products

No matter what the ads on TV spout, soy is NOT a health food at all unless it is fermented. That means natto, miso, and tempeh should be the only soy foods you eat. You can maybe use soy sauce if you don't have problems with gluten All soy sauce contains wheat.

I personally have experienced thyroid problems from consuming soy, thinking that I was eating healthy foods for my body. Nothing could be further from the truth and I have the stack of medical bills to confirm it. Hypothyroidism is becoming epidemic is this country and we need to educate people as to its causes.

The Weston A. Price Foundation (WAP) is an excellent place for doing just that. It is a nonprofit educational foundation that warns the public about the dangers of modern soy foods, in addition to disseminating much other great nutritional information.

The soy story

Here is an introduction by Sally Fallon of WAP to the book *The Whole Soy Story: The Dark Side of America's Favorite Health Food* (New Trends, Spring 2004) written by Kaayla T. Daniels. It can be found at *http://www.westonaprice.org/soy-alert/promotion-of-soy*, or by searching for "Promotion of soy" from the site's homepage. The book is very comprehensive on the subject of soy. Here is a brief quote taken from Sally's introduction:

"'The quickest way to gain product acceptability in the less affluent society,' said a soy-industry spokesperson back in 1975, '...is to have the product consumed on its own merit in a more affluent society.' Thus began the campaign to sell soy products to the upscale consumer, not as a cheap poverty food, but as a miracle substance that would prevent heart disease and cancer, whisk away hot flashes, build strong bones and keep us forever young. ...university professors ...haplessly demonized the competition—meat, milk, cheese, butter and eggs.

Garnering the attention of the health-conscious consumer was an important part of the strategy. Glossy magazines like *Vegetarian Times*, *Health* and *Self* transferred the pro-soy message from health food stores infused with the odor of vitamins to upscale markets, and a raft of books by health professionals encouraged avoidance of meat and dairy as the answer to the rising rates of disease caused by imitation foods.

The funds behind the push for soy are enormous—farmers pay a fee for every bushel of soybeans they sell and a portion of every dollar spent on Twinkies, TV dinners and the thousands of other processed foods that contain soy in one form or another, ultimately go towards the promotion of the most highly processed foods of all—imitation meat, milk, cream, cheese, yogurt, ice cream, candy bars and smoothies made from soy. Even the name of the late Robert Atkins, great defender of beef and butter, has been secunded to the cause. "Low-carb" versions of bread, pastry and pasta—the foods he warned against—are made with high-protein soy."

Soy formula for infants

Soy formula being promoted for infants is especially horrible, in my opinion, and should be outlawed. It is causing premature puberty in both boys and girls, and fertility problems in them too, because of its high estrogen content.

Studies on soy from as early as 1990 show anti-thyroid effects from infants who were fed soy formula, on up to the elderly with goiters and suppressed thyroid function. Concerning these issues, here is another quote from the Weston A Price group which can be found by going to their website at www.westonaprice.org and searching for "Soy Controversy."

"In 1997, scientists Divi, Chang and Doerge of the National Center for Toxicological Research discovered that the antithyroid components in soy were the isoflavones that the industry promotes as panaceas for osteoporosis, heart disease and problems associated with menopause.[13] Low thyroid function can contribute to osteoporosis, heart disease and problems associated with menopause."

Genetically engineered foods

Also, soy is the number one genetically modified food (GMO) on this planet so when you consume it, you are eating "Frankenfoods." There have been no studies done on long term effects on people but problems are beginning to surface in spite of what Monsanto says.

I strongly urge you to educate yourself on all aspects of nutrition so that you can make better decisions as to what you put into your body. Different "experts" have divergent opinions on what constitutes healthy eating and only you can decide what is appropriate for you or your children.

Microwave Ovens

When I first got out of college in 1972 and started working as an adult, the second thing I bought, after a stereo system, was a microwave oven. I remember having an argument with my first husband over whether or not a Thanksgiving turkey cooked in the microwave tasted as good as one cooked the regular way.

It was so much easier and more convenient! I just loved it and used it quite a bit, like so many other people. Little did I know how very dangerous they are.

As with so many other things that are ruining our health, the main stream media refuses to put out any information concerning this. Most people are totally unaware of the hazards of heating things in the microwave.

The hazards of microwave use

One glaring example of this is the nurse in Oklahoma who inadvertently killed a patient. This is from Dr. Mercola's article on the subject:

"In early 1991, word leaked out about a lawsuit in Oklahoma. A woman named Norma Levitt had hip surgery, only to be killed by a simple blood transfusion when a nurse "warmed the blood for the transfusion in a microwave oven"!

Logic suggests that if heating or cooking is all there is to it, then it doesn't matter what mode of heating technology one uses. However, it is quite apparent that there is more to 'heating' with microwaves than we've been led to believe.

Blood for transfusions is routinely warmed - but not in microwave ovens! In the case of Mrs. Levitt, microwaving altered the blood and killed her. Does it not therefore follow that this form of heating does, indeed, do 'something different' to the substances being heated?

Is it not prudent to determine what that 'something different' might do? A funny thing happened on the way to the bank with all that microwave oven revenue: nobody thought about the obvious. Only 'health nuts' who are constantly aware of the value of quality nutrition discerned a problem with the widespread 'denaturing' of our food." *(www.mercola.com/article/microwave/hazards2.htm.)*

Here is a different look at the subject from another page at Dr. Mercola's website:

"It turns out it was the Nazis, who actually invented these ovens. They were used in their mobile support calling them the "radiomissor." These ovens were to be used for the invasion of Russia. By using electronic equipment for preparation of meals on a mass scale, the logistical problem of cooking fuels would have been eliminated, as well as the convenience of producing edible products in a greatly reduced time-factor.

After the war, the Allies discovered medical research done by the Germans on microwave ovens. These documents, along with some working microwave ovens, were transferred to the United States War Department and classified for reference and "further scientific investigation." The Russians had also retrieved some microwave ovens and now have thorough research on their biological effects. As a result, their use was outlawed in the Soviet Union. The Soviets issued an international warning on the health hazards, both biological and environmental, of microwave ovens and similar frequency electronic devices."

How microwave ovens work

The article continues: "All microwave ovens contain a magnetron which is a tube in which electrons are affected by magnetic and electric fields. They produce micro wavelength radiation at about 2450 Mega Hertz (MHz) or 2.45 Giga Hertz (GHz). This microwave radiation interacts with the molecules in food. The wave energy inside the oven changes polarity from positive to negative with each cycle of the wave. These changes happen millions of times every second! Food molecules (especially the molecules of water) have a positive and negative end just like a magnet has a north and a south polarity.

As these microwaves generated from the magnetron bombard the food, they cause the polar molecules to rotate at the same frequency millions of times a second. This is major agitation! (Much less agitation is used in pharmaceutical drug labs to separate or isolate molecules in the making of just about any thing they want.) This agitation creates the molecular friction, which heats up the food. The friction also causes substantial damage to the surrounding molecules, often tearing them apart or forcefully deforming them. The scientific name for this deformation is 'structural isomerism.'" *(http://www.mercola.com/article/microwave/hazards.htm)*

Ten reasons to throw out your microwave oven

"From the conclusions of the Swiss, Russian and German scientific clinical studies, we can no longer ignore the microwave oven sitting in our kitchens. Based on this research, we will conclude this article with the following:

1. Continually eating food processed from a microwave oven causes long term - permanent - brain damage by "shorting out" electrical impulses in the brain [de-polarizing or de-magnetizing the brain tissue].

2. The human body cannot metabolize [break down] the unknown by-products created in microwaved food.

3. Male and female hormone production is shut down and/or altered by continually eating microwaved foods.

4. The effects of microwaved food by-products are residual [long term, permanent] within the human body.

5. Minerals, vitamins, and nutrients of all microwaved food is reduced or altered so that the human body gets little or no benefit, or the human body absorbs altered compounds that cannot be broken down.

6. The minerals in vegetables are altered into cancerous free radicals when cooked in microwave ovens.

7. Microwaved foods cause stomach and intestinal cancerous growths [tumors]. This may explain the rapidly increased rate of colon cancer in America.

8. The prolonged eating of microwaved foods causes cancerous cells to increase in human blood.

9. Continual ingestion of microwaved food causes immune system deficiencies through lymph gland and blood serum alterations.

10. Eating microwaved food causes loss of memory, concentration, emotional instability, and a decrease of intelligence."

(http://www.eutimes.net/2011/02/ten-reasons-to-throw-out-your-microwave-oven)

I strongly encourage you to read all of the aforementioned articles for in-depth facts and figures that show the research behind the hazards of microwave ovens. This information was enough to convince me to never eat anything heated or cooked in a microwave.

Alternatives to microwave ovens

Don't worry, there are alternatives to using a microwave for the three main conveniences. During the winter, I drink hot tea all the time and to keep it warm, I use a plug-in heater and set the cup (ceramic only) on that. It stays toasty warm until the very end. These can be purchased at Amazon if you can't find a local source for one.

Another popular use for a microwave is to pop popcorn. Besides the fact that it is a grain, and as such should not be consumed because it raises your insulin level the same as sugar (see "Grain", page 13), I know that popcorn is very popular. If you want to eat it occasionally, then please pop it on the stove, the old fashioned way.

Stove-top popping really is not that much more difficult to do and you can purchase a specially made pan to do it for you. Mine is from Lehman's *(www.lehmans.com)*, a company that has all kinds of old-fashioned, Amish-type appliances. It's great fun to browse through their website, and it might give you other ideas, too.

The last thing to use instead of a microwave is a hot water appliance for those cups of tea. The "Hot Shot" heater gives you boiling hot water in 30 seconds, quick enough for several mugs at once. Sunbeam makes it, and you can get it at Amazon if you can't find it locally.

Appropriate uses for a microwave

We do still have a microwave in our house, but that is because I am prone to migraine headaches upon occasion. If I can catch the pain in time, I can keep it from becoming a full-blown migraine by putting hot neck warmers on the back of my neck and over my eyes. To warm them up, I use the microwave, but I always stand at least six feet away from it, preferably in the next room, while it's running.

My partner Brian, on the other hand, uses it all the time – to store papers that he wants to hide. That's about the only good use for it. The following was the clincher on it for me.

Microwaves change molecular structure

Dr. Masaru Emoto took pictures of various types of waters and the crystals that they formed. The microwaved water would not form any crystals at all, while the fresh spring water formed beautiful ones. That was the final convincing that I needed.

Dr. Emoto's work was featured in the hit movie *What the Bleep Do We Know?* Further examples of his work can be seen on his web site, which is to be found at *www.masaru-emoto.net/english/entop.html.*

Chapter 3

What To Include

Organic food should top the list of what to include in your diet. What the multi-national, huge conglomerate companies like Monsanto are doing to our food is truly frightening, when you really get down to it. As is discussed in the second chapter, no long-term tests have been done on genetically modified foods at all, and the only way to be sure you're not eating any of those is to eat organic food.

Many people might question why they should eat only organic food, since it is more expensive. If you really value your health and want to optimize it, this is the only way to go.

One other option is to eat locally grown produce so you can get to know the farmers and see for yourself what practices they use. Many use organic methods but are not USDA certified because the process is so expensive and time consuming.

A third option, of course, is to grow your own food so that you can totally control what goes on it and in it. Doing this allows you to be sure your food contains no genetically modified organisms or chemical pesticides.

You will be helping the environment as well by not patronizing CAFOs (Concentrated Animal Feeding Operations) or other big agribusiness atrocities. We vote with our dollars and if no one purchases this type of food, they will have no choice but to go out of business or change their ways.

The Benefits of Organic Food

The Organic Consumers Association has this to say about the difference between conventionally grown and organic foods:

"Organic foods, especially raw or non-processed, contain higher levels of beta carotene, vitamins C, D and E, health-promoting polyphenols, cancer-fighting antioxidants, flavonoids that help ward off heart disease, essential fatty acids, and essential minerals. On average, organic is 25% more nutritious in terms of vitamins and minerals than products derived from industrial agriculture.

Background Information

Since on the average, organic food's shelf price is only 20% higher than chemical food, this makes it actually cheaper, gram for gram, than chemical food, even ignoring the astronomical hidden costs (damage to health, climate, environment, and government subsidies) of industrial food production." *(http://www.organicconsumers.org/organlink.cfm)*

The dangers of conventional farming

The atrocities of our modern day agricultural methods are only getting worse. Dr. Mercola addresses this subject: "The U.S. government is encouraging farmers to spread a chalky waste from coal-fired power plants on their fields to loosen and fertilize soil. The material is produced by power plant "scrubbers" that remove acid-rain-causing sulfur dioxide from plant emissions.

The substance is a synthetic form of the mineral gypsum, and it also contains mercury, arsenic, lead and other heavy metals." *(http://articles.mercola.com/sites/articles/archive/2010/01/16/EPA-Wants-Farmers-to-Spread-Toxic-Coal-Waste-on-Fields.aspx)*

Help is out there!

If your budget is just too tight to buy all of your food organic, then check out this "Dirty Dozen" list of the most pesticide-laden foods and buy those organic. This list can be found at: *http://www.organic.org/articles/showarticle/article-214.*

If you have to buy conventionally grown produce, be aware that the thin-skinned fruits and vegetables (celery, strawberries, peaches, etc.) are the most likely to take up pesticide residue. You can use a mix of vinegar and water to wash lettuce, kale and other leafy greens.

On hard-skinned produce, use running water and a vegetable brush to get off as much as you can. If you are going to soak any of it, be sure to use a swishing motion in the water since it helps to dislodge unwanted things like dirt.

Colleen Huber's article titled "How to Cook Whole Food From Scratch – and Keep your Day Job!" gives you great tips on healthy eating. The article can be found on this web link: *http://articles.mercola.com/sites/articles/archive/2004/05/29/whole-food-cooking.aspx*

And of course, my entire book is geared toward showing you how you can eat healthy on the run and make it fairly easy for you. All it takes is a different mind set and the information that can be found within these pages.

Coconut Oil and Good Fat/Bad Fat

The United States as a nation has been told for the last 40 years to eat a low-fat diet for optimum health. Americans have complied with this dictum in earnest. So why has the rate of obesity skyrocketed to 66% of the population being overweight or obese?

One popular definition of insanity is doing the same thing over and over again expecting different results. I think 40 years is long enough to prove that low-fat diets don't work.

The plain truth of the matter is that fat, as a whole, is your friend. Some fats, namely all trans fats (otherwise known as partially hydrogenated fats), are extremely bad for you and should be avoided at all costs. They are used in a great number of processed foods to prolong shelf life, but do nothing to prolong yours. Be sure to read labels on commercially prepared snack or "junk" foods carefully, or better yet, avoid them altogether.

Fats that are good for you

One of the best oils that you can use is coconut oil. It has a whole host of benefits for your body, both inside and outside. Here is some background information on its history.

The Japanese occupied the Philippines and other South Pacific islands during World War II, effectively shutting off the once plentiful supply of coconut oil to the United States. This oil had long been used as both a cooking oil and an ingredient in numerous food products. Many cookbooks at the turn of the 19th century list it often in their recipes.

To fill the void, American manufacturers began to develop alternative sources of cooking oils — polyunsaturated ones. When the war was finally over, there was a lot of money at stake in the promotion of these vegetable oils. Slick marketing turned public opinion totally against saturated fats like butter and coconut oil, blaming them for raising cholesterol.

The new vegetable oils were erroneously touted as "heart-healthy." To add insult to injury, the soybean industry began to condemn the use of tropical oils, particularly coconut oil, in order to boost their bottom line.

The poorer nations which grew coconuts, like the Philippines and Indonesia, could not counter the negativity spread by rich American industrial conglomerates. Because of this, their economies suffered greatly, as did the health of the people of the United States.

Besides being good for you, using coconut oil would be doing a great service to these developing countries, bolstering them in the manufacturing and exporting of this important oil. They have never quite recovered from the disastrous effects of World War II.

Background Information

Benefits of coconut oil

Most people put all saturated fats in the same category as trans fats, but they are not the same at all. Our parents and grandparents ate butter, lard and coconut oil before WWII and yet there were lower rates of heart disease, diabetes, cancer and obesity than we have today.

Coconut oil is a medium chain triglyceride (MCT) and as such, the body does not handle it in the same way as it does long chain fats, such as vegetable oils. MCTs are smaller and therefore more easily digested, and they are sent straight to the liver to be used for energy instead of being stored as fat. They also raise metabolism and stimulate the thyroid, which can help in weight loss. Coconut oil is high in lauric acid (like mother's milk), and this helps to stimulate the immune system.

This information is from Mary G. Enig, PhD, who is an internationally renowned expert on lipid biochemistry. I will summarize it for you, but if you want further info, the article can be found at the Weston A. Price Foundation *(www.westonaprice.org.)* You can search for it under the title *A New Look at Coconut Oil.*

Dr. Enig found, in a review of the diet/heart disease literature relevant to coconut oil, that the oil is at worst neutral with respect to causing buildup of plaque in arteries. She further ascertained that it is likely to be a beneficial oil for prevention and treatment of some heart disease. Also, coconut oil is a source of anti-microbial fat which can help individuals with compromised immune systems, and it is not a chemical carcinogen.

Medium-chain fats, such as coconut oil, can inactivate bacteria, yeast, fungi, and viruses. Some of the viruses acted upon by these lipids are HIV, measles, and herpes simplex-1, among others. Coconut oil fits the description of a very important functional food.

As you can see from the above, coconut oil is a valuable addition to your diet and the recipes that I offer reflect this. Baked goods are made with coconut oil and coconut flour, and are a delicious alternative to the processed junk that most Americans eat today.

Coconut oil is also the best thing to use in cooking meat, if you want optimal health. It can be used in a frying pan to braise meat, then that meat should be cooked at a low temperature for a longer length of time, for best health as well as taste and tenderness.

The ratio of omega-3 fats to omega-6 fats

Vegetable oils in and of themselves are not bad. However, they are high in omega-6 fats, which are pro-inflammatory in the body, as opposed to omega-3 fats, which are anti-inflammatory. Ideally, the ratio of omega-6s to omega-3s should be 1:1, which is what our ancestors typically consumed.

However the ratio today is closer to 20:1 or even 50:1 which is *way* out of balance, causing too much inflammation and leading to a host of ailments. Organic Extra Virgin Olive Oil, commonly referred to as EVOO, is the best oil to use other than for cooking, as in salads.

One other problem with vegetable oils is that almost all of the most common ones used in products are genetically modified "Frankenfoods." They are soy, canola, cotton seed and corn oils. These oils are found in the majority of processed foods because, since they are subsidized, they are cheap.

If any product says "No trans fats," examine the label carefully. The law states that if the amount per serving is less than 0.5 grams, they can claim "no trans fats." What many companies are doing is lowering the serving size so they can still make that claim. Don't buy anything that has hydrogenated or partially hydrogenated oils.

Changes in omega 3 ratios

Dr. Artemis P. Simopoulos offers valuable information on Omega 3 ratios. He feels that our intake of omega-3 fats is lower today because we don't eat fish as often as we used to. Also, modern industrial animal feeds result in meat that is higher in omega 6 fats. The same is true for eggs and farmed fish. Cultivated vegetables even have fewer omega-3s than their wild counterparts. Overall, the production emphasis of agribusiness has decreased the omega-3 fat content in many foods, including green leafy vegetables, animal meats, eggs, and fish. *(http://articles.mercola.com/sites/articles/archive/2002/04/03/evolution.aspx)*

Excessive consumption of omega-6 fats leads to higher rates of cardiovascular disease, as well as diabetes. Therefore you need to lower the amount of vegetable oils in your diet and raise the amount of omega-3 oils to approximately equal portions.

Another article at Mercola.com has this to say on the subject of omega 6 fats: "Conventionally raised cattle fed corn and soybeans instead of grass become living sources of omega-6 fats. Conversely, free-range chickens that eat grass and bugs lay eggs that contain *10 times* the amount of omega-3 fats than do chickens fed only corn and grains." *(http://blogs.mercola.com/sites/vitalvotes/archive/2006/09/12/new-research-supports-importance-of-lowering-omega-6-fats.aspx)*

Contrary to popular opinion, chickens are not vegetarians and they need to eat bugs. Plus, you get the benefit of great pest control in your gardens.

To continue with another quote from the same article: "Aside from consuming too many omega-6 fats, the other key problem is that many people remain unaware of the problem. Conventional health mainstays like the USDA or the American Heart Association don't talk about the problem or, even worse, don't distinguish between both sets of fats.

Hard to believe such ignorance still exists, especially in light of a new study in today's eHealthy News You Can Use newsletter that found consuming omega-3 fats does a better job of protecting your body from sudden death than a defibrillator can."

That's a pretty strong argument for changing your eating habits to a much more healthy diet. I use the word "diet" in the context of its true definition: how you are going to eat for the rest of your life.

Proper Protein for Shakes

I used to use Pro-Optimal Whey™ from Dr. Mercola in my morning smoothie breakfast drinks. Then he introduced Miracle Whey™ which I felt was better suited to my needs.   I am providing information straight from Dr. Mercola's site about both of these items. You can also search for them by name on his site. Any other protein product that you use is going to have inferior ingredients: sugar or HFCS, pasteurized milk, artificial sweeteners, soy, and/or chemical preservatives.

Pro-Optimal Whey

Pro-Optimal Whey™ is a 100% natural powdered nutrition formula designed to promote peak wellness by optimizing proper protein, fats, carbs and micronutrients. It has no toxic artificial sweeteners or flavors. That means no chemical hazards and no chemical aftertaste. Chocolate and strawberry flavors do contain natural xylitol sweetener, which does not impact blood sugar levels.

The milking cows used to produce Pro-Optimal Whey™ Protein Mix are NEVER subjected to any chemicals, hormones, antibiotics, genetically modified organisms, hyper-immunizations or injected pathogens. The herds graze exclusively on pesticide-free, chemical-free natural grass pastures. Pro-Optimal Whey™ *never* uses cross-flow filtration, micro-filtration, hydrolyzation, ion exchange, or *any* process that could denature the original proteins as found in pure, raw milk. Pro-Optimal Whey™ uses Proserum® Whey Protein. Proserum® is a customized non-denatured, whey protein powder. It undergoes a unique pasteurization process to keep the full range of *all* the fragile immune balancing and restoring components of fresh raw milk.

Plus, these cows are *not* from factory farms that feed their cows grains. Grain-feeding can transform healthy milk proteins into allergens and carcinogens -- which is caused by modern feeding methods that substitute high-protein, soy-based feeds for fresh green grass.

Benefits of Pro-Optimal Whey

Pro-Optimal Whey™ offers prime wellness all in one convenient, economical and delicious drink mix that can help you:

- Balance your blood sugar – ideal for managing hypoglycemia
- Support the health of your liver by aiding in detoxification
- Improve muscle endurance – great for weight training
- Obliterate free radicals with its potent antioxidant properties
- Improve gastrointestinal function and immune system strength with it's immunoglobulins and lactoferrin content.
- Manage your carb intake better with its high protein content and low carbohydrate content

Get ALL the amino acids your body needs – in the best balance yet found in any food, because it contains whey protein and not soy. Pro-Optimal Whey™ is so nutritious it can be used as an alternative to a quick meal.

Miracle Whey™

Dr. Mercola's new Miracle Whey™ has all of the above plus some enhancements to make it even better. There are six flavors to choose from now instead of just three and it is sweetened with Luo Han Guo, a very sweet fruit from China that is powdered and 300 times sweeter than sugar, instead of the Xylitol.

Other whey protein brands

For comparison, I went to my local Kroger store and looked at the ingredient lists of some of the whey protein offered for shakes. Without divulging brand names, here are the lists.

This first brand is actually one of the better offerings out there. Ingredients: cold-processed, cross-flow, microfiltered whey protein isolate, natural flavor, xanthan gum, lecithin, and Stevia. The chocolate brand had the same but with the addition of cocoa powder (natural process).

It's great that they are using Stevia instead of artificial sweeteners but you have to watch out for the term "natural flavorings." Companies do not have to list exactly what is in this due

40

to proprietary laws. They say that if they did, competitors would copy them. However, this is often a cover-up for MSG, which is known by many different names.

The next one had: whey protein concentrate, isomalto-oligosaccharides, cocoa, natural chocolate or vanilla flavoring, sunflower oil, buttermilk, l-leucine, lecithin, dried cream extract, cellulose gum, salt, xanthan gum and sodium alginate.

The last one was the worst: Protein blend (whey and soy), maltodextrin, fructose, sugar, cocoa processed with alkali, rice flour, natural flavor, soy lecithin, medium chain triglycerides, potassium chloride, tricalcium phosphate, salt, ascorbic acid, ferrous fumasate, dicalcium phosphate, vitamin E acetate, niacinamide, zinc oxide, copper gluconate, D-calcium pantothenate, pyroxidine hydrochloride, Vitamin A palmitate, D-biotin, potassium iodide, and cyanocobalamin. (In fairness, most of the last items are the chemical names for added vitamins and minerals.)

I did not check the ingredients for any soy protein products. Just know to always bypass anything containing soy, especially as a main ingredient. Soy lecithin as a later ingredient might be passable. Sugar and fructose are two items you definitely want to avoid for optimal health. I don't know about you, but if something contains so many words that I can't even pronounce, much less know what they mean, I would rather not ingest it.

All About Milk

Real raw milk from free-range, pastured, grass-fed cows is a complete food, containing all 20 amino acids necessary for the human body. It is one of the best sources for healthy natural fats that the human body loves and needs.

Go to the website for Weston A. Price *(www.westonaprice.org)* and search for "transition/dairy" for a page that tells you all about the way the dairy industry has changed the process of selling milk. It has references if you want more information. It is very well done and I strongly recommend that you read it. I will summarize it here, though.

The story of milk

I am one of the Baby Boomers and grew up in the suburbs surrounding Atlanta, Georgia. One of the things I remember my mother saying is, "You know your kids have grown up when you cancel the milk delivery."

Back in those days, fresh milk, cream and half-and-half was delivered directly to your door as often as you ordered it. There was a metal insulated box in which they placed the cold milk and you placed the empty bottles back in after you were finished drinking it. Simple, clean, efficient and no waste to recycle.

We not only survived on this set-up, we thrived on it! As a matter of fact, dairies competed as to who could have the most butterfat in their milk. Can you imagine that? High butterfat was a selling point!

Homogenization

So what happened? To be more competitive, diaries started homogenizing their milk. That way, the fat was distributed evenly throughout the milk and they were all "equal" as far as fat was concerned. Cream did not rise to the top of milk transported in tanker trucks, and so "cheat" some customers out of the butterfat.

It also solved the problem of the dead white cells and bacteria forming sludge on the bottom of the trucks. Homogenization spread the mess evenly throughout the milk so no one would notice it.

In a brilliant coup of advertising, dairies also solved another problem. You see, to make butter, cream and half-and-half, they had to remove the fat from the milk. That gave them all this fat-less milk left over, which was waste material then.

Therefore, they came up with the concept of selling the public on drinking the left-over garbage of non-fat and low-fat milk as a health-promoting product. They could make much more money selling the butter, cream, etc. and make a profit on their waste products, too.

Clever advertising strategy – but there's just one problem. Americans have cut back on fat greatly in the past decades and the rates of obesity have still skyrocketed. So clearly, fat, per se, is not the cause of weight gain. This is discussed in "Good Fat/Bad Fat" (page 35) earlier in this section of the book.

Pasteurization

Homogenization came about after pasteurization. So that dairies in filthy urban places didn't have to clean up their act, they developed pasteurization, a process to destroy bacteria. While this did reduce the rampant diseases that flourished at that time, it could have been accomplished by proper hygiene instead.

Along with killing the bacteria, it destroys many of the vital nutrients that make raw milk so beneficial. Homogenization also causes the cholesterol in the milk to become oxidized, making it rancid and thereby contributing to atherosclerosis and heart disease.

Background Information

The dead bacteria from pus caused by mastitis in the cows (due to eating a diet that is not designed for them) remains in the milk and causes a histamine reaction in susceptible people. The majority of the people who think they are lactose intolerant are really reacting to this dead bacteria and have no problems whatsoever when they switch to raw milk. *(http://www.realmilk.com/untoldstory_1.html.)*

Inhumane agribusinesses

CAFOs (Concentrated Animal Feeding Operations) are horror stories with cows spending their whole adult lives on concrete. They are fed waste products from every conceivable place, from chewing gum past its date (but still in its wrapper), to used oil from restaurants, to leftover parts from slaughterhouses including those of their own species.

They are fed "rendered meat by-products" which consists of road-killed animals and euthanized dogs and cats from vets and animal shelters. These animals may still have their flea collars on and these are thrown in the "pot" with them. Plus they will have the drugs used to put them down still in their bodies. By the way, this is what goes into most commercial pet foods too.

These unnatural foods, along with grains (waste from bakeries) and (usually GMO) soy proteins, change the pH level of the cow's bodies and allow things to go through the intestinal lining that otherwise wouldn't. Therefore they get sick more often and then need antibiotics to control the infections.

Then, of course, there is the synthetic bovine growth hormone (rBGH) that is given to cows to increase their production of milk, again unnaturally. These cows live an average of 42 months as opposed to 12-15 years for those raised on their natural diet of grass. For me, if I can't get raw milk, the least I can do is buy organic so as to minimize the risks and problems for these animals. How we treat our animals is a measure of our "civilization" and right now, that measure is pretty low, in my opinion.

Skim milk is not heart-healthy

One of the worst problems with pasteurization is that the body mounts an immune response, thinking it has been attacked. Not only that, but skim milk has dried milk added to it for "body," to make it palatable. The process used to complete this is sickening, both literally and figuratively.

In *Dirty Secrets of the Food Processing Industry* (which I strongly feel is an absolute MUST READ for everyone!), Sally Fallon states:

"A note on the production of skim milk powder: liquid milk is forced through a tiny hole at high pressure, and then blown out into the air. This causes a lot of nitrates to form and the cholesterol in the milk is oxidized.

Those of you who are familiar with my work know that cholesterol is your best friend; you don't have to worry about natural cholesterol in your food; however, you do not want to eat *oxidized* cholesterol. Oxidized cholesterol contributes to the buildup of plaque in the arteries, to atherosclerosis. So when you drink reduced-fat milk thinking that it will help you avoid heart disease, you are actually consuming oxidized cholesterol, which initiates the process of heart disease." *(www.westonaprice.org—search for "modernfood/dirty-secrets.")*

More on cholesterol

Here is some more information concerning cholesterol that may shed some light on the subject. Remember all those studies that came out that said cholesterol was bad for you?

According to Ray Peat, PhD, "Around 1971, someone noticed that the commercial cholesterol used in feeding experiments was oxidized, that is, it wasn't really cholesterol. Comparing carefully prepared, unoxidized cholesterol with the oxidized degraded material, it was found that pure dietary cholesterol was relatively non-atherogenic." (Source: *Ray Peat's Newsletter September 2005*)

What does this mean? Bruce Fife, N.D., explains, "The cholesterol in fresh milk, eggs and meat is not oxidized and is utilized by the body to strengthen cell membranes, synthesize vital hormones, and build brain and nerve tissue. The drying process in making powdered milk, cheese, and eggs fully oxidizes the cholesterol in these products. Once oxidized it can not be utilized in the normal fashion to build and strengthen body tissues, but is packed away into the plaque of injured arteries. Eating such foods will surely clog your arteries faster than any other substance known on the face of the earth." (Source: *Saturated Fat May Save Your Life*)

Raw milk is superior for your health

One other thing to consider. Fresh raw goat's milk will last two weeks in the refrigerator. After that time it will sour, but will still be good for you to consume if you put some sweetener in it to counteract the sourness. Pasteurized milk past its prime will rot.

A further search of the Weston Price Foundation comes up with this quote: "Pasteurization destroys enzymes, diminishes vitamin content, denatures fragile milk proteins, destroys vitamins C, B12 and B6, kills beneficial bacteria, promotes pathogens and is associated with allergies, increased tooth decay, colic in infants, growth problems in children, osteoporosis, arthritis, heart disease and cancer.

Calves fed pasteurized milk do poorly and many die before maturity. Raw milk sours naturally but pasteurized milk turns putrid; processors must remove slime and pus from pasteurized milk by a process of centrifugal clarification." *(http://www.realmilk.com/what.html)*

I am blessed to have found a great source for raw goat's milk and cow's milk in my local Dawsonville, Georgia area. The state of Georgia allows the sale of raw milk for pet consumption, so for the record, I do have two cats.

There are such things as cow shares and goat shares where you can purchase a "share" in a cow or goat, and then pay the farmer to milk "your" animal. That is perfectly legal, as there are no laws against milking your own cow or goat.

Real Milk--that is, milk that is full fat, unprocessed, and from pasture-fed cows or goats is the way to go. Please do NOT consume raw milk from conventional confinement dairies or dairies which produce milk intended for pasteurization.

Real Milk, produced under clean conditions and promptly refrigerated, contains many anti-microbial and immune-supporting components. This protective system in raw milk can be overwhelmed, and the milk contaminated, in situations where the seller does not follow healthy hygiene protocols.

The bottom line is, know your farmer! I will be happy to give any of my local Dawsonville readers the information on where I get my raw goat's and cow's milk. I use it to make yogurt and kefir, both fermented items with great health benefits.

Questions about casein

One last concern to address is the question of casein. All milk has casein in it. Some of it is A1 casein, and some of it is A2, depending on the breed of mammal (and sometimes the specific animal within that breed). A1 casein has been associated with Type 1 diabetes, autism, schizophrenia and heart disease. A2 casein has been shown to do the opposite. All goat's milk contains A2 casein and therefore is never a problem. You can Google this for more information.

Alternatives for Vegans or Vegetarians

If you are vegetarian or vegan, you can use coconut milk, almond milk or rice milk, all of which should be organic. The coconut milk, unless you buy fresh coconuts, may be in cans, which carry their own problems, notably BPA (Bisphenol A, a carcinogen) in the linings and lids. Now it is being sold in cartons just like regular milk and that is a better option. The almond milk will be not raw, despite the label (see information below on that topic.)

The FDA has just approved genetically modified rice so always buy organic on that. You can get around the cooked almonds by buying them direct from the growers and thus eliminating the middle men who by law have to irradiate or cook them. Then you can make your own almond milk with the recipe on page 52 of this book.

Essential news about raw almonds

Here is some valuable information about almonds, from D and S Ranches of California:

"Important News About Our Shippable Almond Crop!

D&S Ranches, an Orchard Grower in the San Joaquin Valley of California, has an Important Announcement to make regarding Pasteurization of our Naturally Grown California Almonds! After the Almond Board Rule went into effect we began to extensively research the Best, most Non-Intrusive methods available to reduce bacteria on the skin of the nut without affecting the nut meat itself.

The Good News:

The Good news is that we have found a process that does just that! This method was developed for the Spices Food Group where any alteration or destruction of the interior of the nut or spice kernel would destroy the delicate value of the item. As it turns out we were able to get this technology approved for application on our Selma California Grown Nut Crop!

How It Works:

- The process is very expensive and requires the latest in production technology. It is centered on Water Based Botanical Principles. We call this process H20-UN-Pasteurization. The almonds are held in a chamber that draws down the air to a vacuum, so all the air born [sic] bacteria and pathogens are removed from the chamber, then a computer controlled mist of sterile distilled water dry steam is injected in to the chamber. This steam is computer controlled and balanced against the known weight of each nut. As the small amount of steam condenses on the skin of the nut it transfers only minimal heat energy just to the surface it contacts! The nut meat is never heated internally!

- After the dry steam injection, a 4 to 6 second process, the chamber is then evacuated again causing the condensed purified water to evaporate from the skin of the nut. Next the chamber is brought back to normal conditions with HEPA Filtered Air.

- This process preserves the internal natural balance of enzymes, amino acids, proteins, and most importantly it preserves the natural living nature of the nut! You can sprout these Almonds!

- We are sure you will be very satisfied with this process, and as far as we know we are the only Ranch Direct Almond Grower in the San Joaquian Valley of California that is using this expensive, and time consuming process, so that we may bring you the very finest in US Graded Fancy #1 California Almonds!

Please beware of other processes:

We are concerned that there are a good number of other processes out there that are very inferior and some are outright dangerous! The most common is simple autoclave sterilization and this is, essentially, just cooking the nut. After an autoclave process, the nut is no longer living, it is dead, and all the valuable nutrients of the nut have been cooked and destroyed. Unfortunately the Almond Board, under presser from the Big Almonds Handlers, Processors and Growers are calling and labeling, in the stores, these nuts as RAW! They ARE NOT RAW! They are COOKED!

Other processes are using PPO (Propylene Oxide Gas). You should never, ever under any circumstances eat nuts exposed to PPO Gas. PPO is a known carcinogen (causes cancer). It is toxic and poisonous! The European Union (EU) has prohibited the use of PPO Gas on any Human Food Product. The USDA and the FDA still allow it. Inquire with your store if their nuts have been exposed to PPO! Make sure you know! This is serious business."

Please go to D and S Ranches for more information on purchasing truly raw almonds, or go to *www.livingtreecommunity.com*.

Order nuts directly from the growers online

You may purchase these almonds directly from the growers by accessing their web site above. You can purchase them in bulk and share with your neighbors and friends for the best deal. See *Soaking nuts, grains and fruits* under "Raw Foods Guidelines" on page 6 for additional information about optimal health from these sources.

Whatever you choose, please continue to support our American farmers, who are trying to find alternative ways to process almonds so that they will not be hit with a recall of bacteria laden almonds that would just devastate them and put them out of business.

How to Make Yogurt

Consuming yogurt is extremely beneficial for you on your quest for healthy eating. Anything that you buy in the store is going to be pasteurized by law so it is best to make your own. Plus it is very easy to do!

Yogurt can be made from raw goat or cow's milk, if that is available to you, or from coconut milk, if you are vegetarian or vegan. I use a Yolife yogurt maker from Tribest which has seven small ½ cup jars with lids so that you can have one for each day of the week.

This particular brand also has a large lid that you can use to make yogurt in bigger containers. Only use a non-metal utensil to stir the yogurt. I use a wire whisk covered in non-scratch material and mix until the yogurt from the store is distributed throughout. For some reason, metal does not work well with yogurt and may cause it to not form properly.

Get live active cultures

I add three heaping tablespoons of store-bought, plain yogurt to my milk when making the yogurt. Make sure that whatever brand you buy says, "Live active cultures." It's not enough for it to say "contains bacteria." (These are probiotics, or helpful bacteria, that beneficially populate our intestines to aid digestion. The more you have the merrier.) Also be sure the yogurt you buy is not sweetened, and is preferably made from goat's milk.

By the way, our gut constitutes 80% of our immune system. We want to have 85% good bacteria to 15% of the bad guys for a healthy system. That's why I use my milk raw, as heating it destroys these beneficial bacteria.

How to make the yogurt

The first thing I do when making yogurt is to sterilize the large and small containers with boiling water. After that, set the containers in the bottom part of the yogurt maker.

When you pour the milk into the containers, only pour it to the top bend in the jar at first. Sometimes the yogurt settles to the bottom of the mixing bowl so save the last bit and pour it into each of the jars at the end to fill them up completely. This ensures that the yogurt culture is added fairly equally to each jar.

After filling the jars, DO NOT put the lids on them. Add the top cover just barely fitting onto the bottom and plug it in. Mark the time on the top dial and let it sit for eight to twelve hours (overnight works great).

Finishing up the yogurt

When the yogurt is finished, take the lid off as carefully as you can to prevent condensation from falling into the yogurt. If it does, no harm is done; it just makes the yogurt more watery. If the yogurt has set up properly, it should be creamy and yummy just like the original.

Once you have the top cover off, put the lids on the jars and store them in the refrigerator (unless you want to indulge in some warm yogurt over fruit right then and there). Since it is plain yogurt, you will want to add your natural sweetener of choice: Stevia, Luo Han Guo (find it on-line) or Xylitol. I prefer Stevia or Lo Han.

I use a food grade plastic spoon that I purchased from a camping supply store whenever I eat the yogurt or spoon it out. It's best to avoid fast food cutlery just on general principles. For pictures of this process, go to my website at *www.HealthyEatingOnTheRun.com/how-to-make-yogurt.html*.

Yogurt starters

You can add more or less yogurt "starter" (the plain store-bought yogurt) at the beginning, to your taste. You may also purchase yogurt starter cultures alone from Hoegger Goat Supply online if you prefer (see their website at *www.hoeggergoatsupply.com*.) That way you won't have the problem of using pasteurized products.

The Hoegger starter only has three different kinds of probiotics. Although pasteurized, Cascade Fresh brand yogurt at Whole Foods has eight separate probiotics. To be active, the bacteria are added after the milk is pasteurized, therefore it's okay to use if you can't get anything else.

Goat's milk yogurt from Redwood Hill Farms is a great one to use, too. Goat's milk yogurt is not homogenized because it doesn't need to be. Organic markets will likely carry goat's milk yogurt so you can keep the kind of milk the same, if possible. This is ideal, but the goat's milk yogurt is somewhat pricey.

Be aware that the cow's milk used to make commercial yogurt is homogenized, which is not good for you (see "All About Milk" on page 40). It's always a trade off if you can't get raw milk during the winter time.

Use it for five "generations"

You can use your last jar of homemade yogurt to start your new batch the next time. This can be done for up to five "generations" of yogurt, basically four times after the initial batch. There is a kind of natural bacteria in milk that keeps it fresh.

Try adding fruit to your yogurt. I sometimes use yogurt in my Morning Wake Up Shake, adding the sweetener just before I drink my smoothie, not right after making the yogurt. I also use yogurt on my homemade Sweet Breakfast Granola, which I eat as a dessert or snack sometimes. I occasionally add fresh fruit in season to that, too. Be creative and try your yogurt on lots of things!

Cultured or fermented foods are extremely beneficial for optimum health. See "All About Milk" on page 40 for further info.

Alternative method of making yogurt

There is an article on *About.com* that details six ways to make yogurt without a yogurt maker. It includes methods for making it in a thermos, an oven, a heating pad, in the sun, on a wood stove, and in a crockpot. Details can be found here: *http://homecooking.about.com/od/dairyrecipes/r/bldairy9.htm?p=1*. You can also make yogurt in a dehydrator, or a small six-pack cooler. Your dehydrator should have instructions included in the manual.

Here is some information on the cooler method: First, sterilize two pint jars. Heat four cups of milk until a clean knuckle inserted into it feels neutral, neither hot nor cold. Then add about a tablespoon of yogurt starter (plain, not sweetened) to each jar, using a non-metal spoon. Pour half of the warm milk into each jar. Do not stir.

Place the uncovered jars into the cooler and pour hot, but not boiling, water into it around the jars, to within one inch of the top of the jars. Close the lid of the cooler and set it where it won't be disturbed. Leave the jars in the cooler for at least eight hours (up to about ten), then put the lids on, and store them in the refrigerator. There may be some whey on top, or if using raw cow's milk, maybe some cream.

Add a sweetener of your choice to each serving when you spoon it out of the container. You can also save a little to use as your next starter batch, up to five "generations."

Making Kefir

There are two different kinds of kefir that you can make: sugar water kefir and milk kefir. Making either is a lot more challenging than making yogurt, but especially the water kefir.

You have to purchase starter grains, kind of like making sourdough bread, and you have to take care of the grains (which reproduce themselves), and find other folks to give them to, or discard them.

Water kefir tastes absolutely wonderful and has lots of probiotics, but it also contains sugar, which you ideally want to avoid. Do not try making it with anything else like stevia or xylitol. I tried it and it tasted awful, plus I had to throw out the grains afterwards.

It also requires attention every 48 hours and you can't miss it or the grains go bad. You have to drink it fairly quickly, too, because it will not keep very long. Even though I liked it very much, I was gaining weight with all the sugar and was spending way too much time on it, so I gave it up.

Making water kefir

If you want to try making some of the sugar water kefir on your own, I will refer you to Dom's web site at: *http://users.sa.chariot.net.au/~dna/kefirpage.html*. He is the undisputed King of Kefir and is located in Australia. You can get the grains from a source here in the United States through the mail.

I do agree with Dom that milk kefir should be made with raw milk to be optimally beneficial for you. You can buy Lifeway brand commercially-made kefir from most grocery stores. However, it is pasteurized, usually low-fat, and has sugar in it, so I don't recommend it for those reasons.

Making milk kefir

Making your own milk kefir at home is fairly straightforward and using the natural grains is best for your health. You will have to go to Dom's site to order the grains. Again, you have to be diligent about keeping up with it, and that gets to be a drain after awhile.

So, I have opted to use starter grains that I purchase from Dr. Mercola's web site. For my Georgia readers, you may purchase them closer to home from the Hoegger's Goat Supply web site at *www.hoeggergoatsupply.com* They are a local Georgia company located in Fayetteville. I try to support local people whenever possible.

Once you make a batch of kefir, you keep out six tablespoons of "starter" for the next batch, and you can repeat this for a total of seven generations. Then it's time to get a new batch. It's best to start a new batch within three days of finishing the old one.

Of course, some people may be asking, "Why go to all this trouble"? Why indeed? Dr. Weston A. Price, in his groundbreaking book *Nutrition and Physical Degeneration*, points out that ALL of the healthiest native tribes that he studied ate fermented foods of some kind. That was the common denominator among all of them.

Fermented food

It is vitally important that we add some kind of fermented food to our diets if we want to have optimum health. Sally Fallon Morell and Mary G. Enig wrote a very informative article on this subject. Here is an excerpt:

"Acid porridges made from grains are far superior to western grain preparations. Fermentation increases mineral availability by neutralizing phytic acid, increases vitamin content, predigests starches and neutralizes enzyme inhibitors. Insoluble fiber can cause pathogenic changes in the intestinal tract unless properly soaked in an acid medium.[9] Oat bran, which is high in phytic acid, as well as related bran products can cause numerous problems with digestion and assimilation, leading to mineral deficiencies, irritable bowel syndrome and autoimmune difficulties such as Crohn's disease. Case control studies indicate that consumption of cereal fiber can be linked with *detrimental* effects on colon cancer formation.[10]" *(http://www.westonaprice.org/traditional_diets/out_of_africa.html)*

The authors went on to say that fermented foods had a significant impact on products of digestion, bringing transit time and elimination back to optimal levels. From this, you can see that yogurt and kefir are the two products that will help those of us who eat a Western diet the most. Of those two, yogurt is the easier to obtain and to make yourself, but kefir has its benefits, too.

Instructions for making milk kefir

If you want to try making this type of kefir, here are the instructions:

1. Sterilize the container in which you will culture your kefir with boiling water. A glass jar that can be closed is best, but any container with a lid will do.
2. Using a glass or enameled pot, heat one quart of milk (or two cups if using goat's milk) over medium-low heat for about five minutes. Slowly and gently bring it up to skin temperature (about 92° F).
3. Stick a clean knuckle into it until it feels neutral, neither hot nor cold, to the touch. The idea is to heat it gently to maintain all the good bacteria and enzymes.
4. Remove from heat.
5. Add the starter package to it, using non-metal utensils.

6.   Stir until the ferment has dissolved completely.

7.   Pour the inoculated milk into the jar and close the lid.

8.   Ferment the mixture at between 72°-75° F for 18-24 hours in a place where it will not be disturbed. The top of a refrigerator is a good choice.

9.   The mixture will thicken and turn slightly lumpy, and will have a distinct sour smell to it. It will turn milky white and may have some bubbles form on top. The taste will be slightly tart and tangy and little of the original sweetness will remain.

10. Refrigerate after fermentation. It will continue to ferment but at a slower pace.

11. Save six tablespoons of the culture to start the next batch. This may be done for seven generations before discontinuing and using a new starter packet the next time.

It is best to start the next new batch within three days. Batches will last approximately one week in the refrigerator. The lactic acid generated by the fermentation process acts as a preservative. The milk sugar (lactose) wakes up the bacteria in the starter, which then feed on and grow in the milk. This creates beneficial probiotics which are essential for good intestinal floral health.

You may sweeten your kefir with the natural sweetener of your choice: Stevia, Luo Han Guo, or xylitol. The kefir culture starter can be stored in the refrigerator for at least 18 months. Now that you have made your kefir, you can use it in the Morning Wake Up Shake, the Sweet Breakfast Granola, or just over fruit as a snack. The probiotics will greatly aid in digestion.

Making Almond Milk

If you are vegan or just prefer not to consume dairy products, here is a recipe for making almond milk that you can use over cereal or as desired. You can leave the skins on the almonds. They will not harm you, but do leave little pieces in the milk (which is not very attractive).

Therefore, you may prefer to take the skins off of the almonds, which results in a white looking liquid that resembles thin cow's milk or skim milk. Removing the skins does involve a bit of work, although kids usually find it fun, at least the first time.

Before you start, you need to soak the almonds for 8-10 hours (overnight is ideal). Nuts are soaked to remove the enzyme inhibitors from them, so always pour off the soaking water when finished.

Enzyme inhibitors are on all seeds to keep them safe until the conditions are right for them to grow. These conditions are light, warmth, and water, usually with soil included too, except in the case of hydroponics.

Getting the skins off the almonds

1. Take the soaked almonds and put them in an enamel or metal (non-glass) bowl.
2. Heat water in a separate pan until boiling.
3. Pour the boiling water over the almonds and stir them for about a minute, no longer, because you don't want to cook them.
4. Immediately transfer the almonds into cold water. The skins should come off easily but if they don't, repeat the process.
5. Take off the skins by holding them between the thumb and index finger and pushing on the skin. Be careful, as they have a tendency to shoot across the room!

And there you have it! White almonds.

Making plain almond milk

1 cup of almonds, skins off if preferred
3 cups of good filtered water

1. Put the almonds into the Vita-mix with 1½ cups of filtered or well water and blend until smooth.
2. Then add another 1½ cups of water and continue blending.

This will leave you with a somewhat chunky kind of milk. If the pieces of almonds are a problem, blend them further, or strain them out of the milk through cheesecloth or a fine strainer.

Making sweet almond milk

1 cup almonds, with or without skins
3 cups good filtered water
1 teaspoon Vanilla Extract
a dash of Stevia or Luo Han Guo to taste

Process as for the plain recipe. Add the sweetener and vanilla after the water, but while still blending.

Making yogurt from almond milk

If you so desire, you can make yogurt from almond milk, too. (I personally don't care for the consistency.) You can use the cultures as listed in **"How to Make Yogurt"** page 48, or take two or three probiotic capsules per blender-full and break them into the blender.

Use the Yolife yogurt maker the same way you would for other milk. Or if you don't have a yogurt maker, you can pour the contents into a non-metal bowl and let it sit out on the counter, covered, for five to eight hours at room temperature.

Taste it after five or six hours to see if it's slightly sour, because when it is sour, it is finished. The more sour it is, the more cultured it is, but it is up to your individual taste.

Add the sweetener of your choice (see "Natural Sweeteners" page 55 in this section) and maybe some vanilla if desired. Use it over cereal, with fruit, or in a smoothie, the same way you would use other types of yogurt.

See "How to Make Yogurt" page 47 for more information on ways to make yogurt. There is information about raw almonds in the same section.

These almonds may be purchased directly from the growers by accessing their web site at *http://www.almonds-from-california.com*. You can purchase them in bulk and share with your neighbors and friends for the best deal.

Salba™ and Chia Seeds

Salba is a relatively unknown powerhouse seed found in South America. The Aztec Indians referred to it as their "running food" because it gave them such amazing energy and power. Runners relaying messages relied on it as their sole source of nourishment while delivering these communications.

Gram for gram, it has 8 times more omega-3s than salmon, 1.1 times more fiber than all types of bran, 15 times more magnesium than broccoli, 30% more antioxidants than blueberries, 3 times more iron than spinach and 6 times more calcium than milk. Plus, it has both soluble and insoluble fiber and it is a complete vegetable protein.

Adding Salba to your diet can help with digestive problems (bloating, diarrhea, and constipation), support a healthy cardiovascular system, alleviate joint stiffness, regulate blood sugar, and give you more energy. It has over 30 different nutrients in their whole food form, which makes them more bioavailable to the body.

Web site info

Here's what the web site *"Salba – The Salba Group"* has to say about it: "Today, experts say Salba is the most nutritionally complete food in nature. It's the richest plant-based source of Omega-3 fatty acids, has the highest protein content of any seed or grain, is loaded with both soluble and insoluble fiber, and contains high levels of antioxidants, calcium, magnesium and iron."

Salba can currently be purchased at some local grocers, as well as organic markets. You can also buy chia seeds, which are much less expensive but are also less nutritious for you. The chia seeds are the brown ones mixed in with the white ones with many more of the brown than the white ones. Getting only the white ones is what makes the Salba seeds so much more expensive. Either one would be a very good addition to a healthy diet.

Natural Sweeteners

You'll be happy to know that there are several alternative sweeteners that you can use to prepare foods and not miss your just desserts in life. I have done my share of going to the refrigerator, opening the door and just staring inside, waiting for something to call to me.

What did I want? Something sweet? No, I tried a cookie and wasn't satisfied. Something salty? Nope, I ate chips and still had a craving. Something fatty (my usual downfall)? No, I tried some cheese and that didn't work either.

Finally I figured out that what I wanted was not food, but rather, comfort, and no kind of food was going to give me that. Once I finally got over my physical cravings for various types of food (and that was a long journey), I realized that what I wanted was some sweetness in my life.

I'm a very disciplined person and I was working way too much and taking no time for myself. So even though I wasn't physically craving sweets, I did want a little taste of something sweet to finish out my meal. Usually I needed to get the strong taste of garlic and onions off my breath, too, as I do eat a lot of those.

Therefore I do feel that it is important to have some sweetness in our lives, and there are many desserts that can be made that are actually good for you. So you can relax now and breathe easier. Healthy eating can even be fun!

56

Xylitol

You have probably never heard of this sweetener but it is great for use in baking as a substitute for sugar. It gives baked goods more body since you use it measure for measure the same way you use sugar.

Xylitol is a sugar alcohol that is naturally found in strawberries, birch bark and corn cobs. This is from the web site *www.xylitol.org* which has this to say: "Xylitol is right here, inside, already. Our bodies produce up to 15 grams of xylitol from other food sources using established energy pathways. Xylitol is not a strange or artificial substance, but a normal part of everyday metabolism.

Xylitol is widely distributed throughout nature in small amounts. Some of the best sources are fruits, berries, mushrooms, lettuce, hardwoods, and corn cobs. One cup of raspberries contains less than one gram of xylitol."

From the web site *www.xylitolinfo.com* comes this: "Xylitol is a low-glycaemic sweetener and is metabolized independently of insulin. Xylitol does not cause the sharp increase in blood sugar levels or the associated serum insulin response, which is usually seen following consumption of other carbohydrates. Thus, Xylitol can be recommended as a sugar-free sweetener suitable for diabetics as well as for the general population seeking a healthier lifestyle."

For a little bit of the history of Xylitol, this is from Emerald Forest brand's brochure: "During World War II, Finland was suffering from a sugar shortage and with no domestic supply of sugar, they searched for, and rediscovered, an alternative – xylitol. It was only when xylitol was stabilized that it became a viable sweetener in foods."

Many of my baked recipes include the use of Xylitol so it will be referenced many times in the creation of breads and desserts. One slight caution though: if you consume too much of it at one time, it can have a slight laxative effect. This will resolve as the body's enzymatic activity adjusts. Therefore, use all things in moderation.

Stevia

I am in complete agreement with Dr. Mercola on the best sweetener for everyday use. He advocates Stevia, explaining as follows:

"Unlike aspartame, sucralose and other artificial sweeteners that have been cited for dangerous toxicities, stevia is a natural alternative that's ideal for diabetics, those watching their weight and anyone interested in maintaining their health. Stevia can be used in appetizers, beverages, soups, salads, vegetables, desserts -- virtually anything! It is, hands down, the best alternative to sugar you will ever taste." *(http://articles.mercola.com/sites/articles/archive/2004/12/29/splenda-equal.aspx)*

Stevia is the sweetener I use most often in a number of my deserts, along with my Sweet Breakfast Granola. It is 200-300 times sweeter than sugar so a little bit goes a very long way. For a comparison, you can go to my website *www.HealthyEatingOnTheRun.com.natural-sweeteners.html,* to the page on Natural Sweeteners, and take note of the size of the "spoon" included with this brand of Stevia. Use that as your guide.

Both Stevia and Xylitol could previously be found only in the supplement section of stores, not in the sweetener section. At my Kroger, it is up front in the Natural Market (organic) section of the store.

Perhaps now that some of the big manufacturers are starting to use Stevia combined with erythritol, some even combining it with sugar, the FDA will reverse its idiotic stance that Stevia is unsafe to be used by itself. This has been done in capitulation to the artificial sweetener industry and has resulted in confiscation of both produce and books in the past, totally unfairly in my opinion.

I'm also seeing a few companies coming out with pure Stevia in packets, so I think that's a step in the right direction, too.

Luo Han Guo

There's a good chance you have never heard of this product, either, but it is a marvelous natural sweetener. From Dr. Ray Sahelian's site I quote this:

LUO HAN GUO fruit by Ray Sahelian, M.D.

"Luo han guo is a very sweet fruit found in China. Extracts of luo han guo (also spelled Luo han kuo, or lo han kuo) are now being marketed as a sweetener. The amounts normally used are so small that luo han guo is not likely to have any appreciable effect on human physiology.

My [Dr. Sahelian's] experience with luo han guo

I keep luo han guo on my kitchen counter and use it to sweeten teas. It is low-calorie, has a fruity sweetness, and I would recommend it as an alternative to sugar and artificial sweeteners." *(raysahelian.com)*

It's great that we now have these low or no-calorie alternatives to traditional sweeteners: Stevia and Luo Han Guo. I prefer Lo Han in my teas, especially.

Lo Han Sweet Jarrow Formulas

The following is taken from the Jarrow Formulas (a California-based manufacturer of Lo Han) website: "Lo Han Kuo is the fruit of Momordica grosvenori, a plant cultivated in the mountains of southern China. Mogrosides, which are water extracted from the Lo Han fruit, offer a pleasant, sweet taste without elevating blood sugar. Lo Han Kuo Mogrosides are up to 250x sweeter than sugar.

Xylitol, a naturally occurring polyol, is sweet with a distinct cooling sensation in the mouth. Xylitol is metabolized differently from a conventional sugar and does not cause or contribute to tooth decay. Xylitol is as sweet as sugar, having 40% less calories.

Lo Han Sweet advantages:

Low Glycemic Index: Does not cause extreme fluctuations in blood sugar.

Heat Stable: Very stable under high temperature, and can be added to both hot as well as cold foods. Suitable for cooking and baking."

I have not been able to find any local sources for this and my supply was given to me by a friend, but if you go online, you can buy it from several places there. Jarrow brand is one company that carries it as well as Body Ecology. I go back and forth between Stevia and Luo Han Guo for variety.

Agave Nectar

This is an article from Dr. Mercola's website explaining his views on agave: "Many varieties of agave nectar are processed at relatively low temperatures (below 118°F) and are marketed as a "raw" food.

The Myth of Agave as a "Healthy" Sugar Substitute

- Agave syrup is neither a natural food nor organic

Fully chemically processed sap from the agave plant is known as hydrolyzed high fructose inulin syrup. According to Dr. Ingrid Kohlstadt, a fellow of the American College of Nutrition and an associate faculty member at Johns Hopkins School of Public Health:

'[Agave is] almost all fructose, highly processed sugar with great marketing.'

- Agave syrup is not low calorie.
- Agave syrup is about 16 calories per teaspoon, the same as table sugar.
- Agave syrup may not have a low glycemic index.

Depending upon where the agave comes from and the amount of heat used to process it, your agave syrup can be anywhere from 55% to 90% fructose! (And it's likely you won't be able to tell from the product label.) This range of fructose content hardly makes agave syrup a logical choice if you're hoping to avoid the high levels of fructose in HFCS (high fructose corn syrup).

And if you're diabetic, you should know that the alleged benefit of agave for diabetics is purely speculative. Very few agave studies have been documented, and most involved rats. There have been no clinical studies done on its safety for diabetics.

Since most agave syrup has such a high percentage of fructose, your blood sugar will likely spike just as it would if you were consuming regular sugar or HFCS, and you would also run the risk of raising your triglyceride levels. It's also important to understand that whereas the glucose in other sugars are converted to blood glucose, fructose is a relatively unregulated source of fuel that your liver converts to fat and cholesterol.

A significant danger here is that fructose does not stimulate your insulin secretion, nor enhance leptin production, which is thought to be involved in appetite regulation. (This was detailed in one of the most thorough scientific analyses published to date on this topic.). . . dietary fructose can also contribute to increased food intake and weight gain. Therefore, if you need to lose weight, fructose is one type of sugar you'll definitely want to avoid, no matter what the source is.

Other dangers of fructose

In addition, consuming high amounts of concentrated fructose may cause health problems ranging from mineral depletion, to insulin resistance, high blood pressure, cardiovascular disease, and even miscarriage in pregnant women.

Fructose may also interfere with your body's ability to metabolize copper. This can result in depletion of collagen and elastin, which are vital connective tissues. A copper deficiency can also result in anemia, fragile bones, defects in your arteries, infertility, high cholesterol and heart disease, and uncontrolled blood sugar levels.

Additionally, fructose consumption has been shown to significantly increase uric acid. Elevated levels of uric acid are markers for heart disease. It has also been shown to increase blood lactic acid, especially in diabetics. Elevations in lactic acid can result in metabolic acidosis.

Isolated fructose has no enzymes, vitamins or minerals and can rob your body of these nutrients in order to assimilate itself. Hence, consumption of fructose can also lead to loss of vital minerals like calcium, iron, magnesium, and zinc.

Background Information

Other reasons you should steer clear of agave

1. There are very few quality controls in place to monitor the production of agave syrup. Nearly all agave sold in the U.S. comes from Mexico. Industry insiders are concerned agave distributors are using lesser, even toxic, agave plants due to a shortage of blue agave.

    There are also concerns that some distributors are cutting agave syrup with corn syrup—how often and to what extent is anyone's guess. In addition, the FDA has refused shipments of agave syrup due to excessive pesticide residues.

2. Agave syrup is not a whole food—it is fractionated and processed. The sap is separated from the plant and treated with heat, similar to how maple sap is made into maple syrup. Agave nectar is devoid of many of the nutrients contained in the original, whole plant.

3. Agave syrup is not a live food. The natural enzymes are removed to prevent agave syrup from fermenting and turning into tequila in your food pantry or cabinet.

4. Agave is, for all intents and purposes, highly concentrated sugar. Sugar and sweeteners wreak havoc on your health and are highly addictive." *(http://blogs.mercola.com/ sites/vitalvotes/archive/2009/06/16/agave-a-triumph-of-marketing-over-truth.aspx)*

On a personal note, I have tried agave nectar and it gave me horrendous headaches, so I definitely will not use it. It is your choice if you want to try it, but with all of this information, I would avoid it just on general principles.

Please refer back to page 52 on high fructose corn syrup. Though it is made from corn, a substance found in nature, it is not something that should be eaten at all, for many reasons.

The fructose naturally found in fruits is perfectly fine to ingest, especially if you eat the whole fruit instead of only the juice. That way, you get much-needed fiber and your body gets a feeling of fullness instead of sensing it as hydration only.

Chapter 4

What's Your Beef? (and Eggs)

Grass-fed, Grass-finished Beef

Most of the meat eaten in the United States comes from CAFOs (Concentrated Animal Feeding Operations) which are, in my opinion, grossly inhumane ways of treating animals. The problems they cause are many, not the least of which is the horrendous accumulation of waste material.

In pastured animal operations, the ground can readily handle the animal's manure and it actually enriches it. But when you have mountains of manure, it goes into the local waterways and underground streams and overwhelms them.

These CAFOs feed their animals grains, and other atrocious things (see "All About Milk," page 40, in the previous chapter for more details), and most of the grains are genetically modified. So, we have no idea what long-term effects this may have on the human body.

On the subject of cattle, grass-fed is absolutely the winner. Dr. Mercola has this to say: "... scientific experiments determined that if the ratio of omega 6 fats to omega 3 fats exceeds 4:1, people have more health problems. This is especially meaningful since grain-fed beef can have ratios that exceed 20:1 whereby grass-fed beef is down around 3:1.

Similar ratios are also found in all grain-fed versus grass-fed livestock products. Grassfed products are rich in all the fats now proven to be health-enhancing, but low in the fats that have been linked with disease." *http://www.mercola.com/beef/health_benefits.htm*

In another article, he states that: "Several studies point to the health benefits of grass-fed beef, as distinguished from cattle raised on corn-based feed. In addition to having higher levels of "good fats" such as omega-3's and conjugated linoleic acids (CLAs), grass-fed beef has significantly less fat and far fewer calories.

Grass-fed beef also avoids some of the health concerns associated with cattle fed on grain. The outbreak of mad cow disease in Europe in the 1990s was caused by grain that was mixed with meat-and-bonemeal from contaminated cows." *http://blogs.mercola.com/sites/vital*

votes/archive/2008/08/01/grass-fed-beef-is-better-for-your-health-and-the-environment.aspx.

Be aware that many companies label their beef "grass-fed" and there is no oversight for that usage. All beef can be classified that way in that, after weaning, the calves do graze on grass until they reach a certain size.

Then two months before they are ready for slaughter, they feed them corn to fatten them up. "Grass-finished" is the term you need to look for, to avoid any corn feeding.

The best grass-fed, grass-finished beef around

For us in the South, the very best company to find this at is Whiteoak Pastures in South Georgia. They not only graze their animals their whole lives, but they recently built their own slaughterhouse so that their cows would not be traumatized by being trucked far away.

They also use all parts of the cow in their ground beef so that you might be getting steak or filet mignon in with it. It is absolutely superb tasting and saves you the cost of buying expensive steaks. Please take the time to check out their operations and view their new video documentary "Cud," done by the Southern Foodways Alliance in the summer of 2009. It's on their great website, found at *http://www.whiteoakpastures.com/*.

For my local Dawsonville readers, Wrights' Farm in Ellijay is the best for the same type of beef, plus heritage pork, eggs and milk. See page 64 for more in-depth information.

The difference between white meat and dark meat

Concerning poultry, here is some information from Dr. Mercola on the differences between white and dark meat.

"Confused about what makes white meat "white" and dark meat "dark"? You're not alone. Misleading data about the good and bad sides of white and dark meat abound. Finally, here is the real truth about the meat you eat.

Dark Meat

Simply speaking, dark meats are dark because the muscles are used more (think drumsticks vs. breast meat). They have more myoglobin proteins, which help ship oxygen to your muscle cells.

When dark meat is cooked, the myoglobins turn into metmyoglobins, which are very high in iron.

White Meat

White meat contains glycogen, which is a polysaccharide of glucose, an animal starch. Animal starch is stored in your liver, then broken down into glucose when it's needed by the white muscle.

Nutritional Differences

Dark meat contains more zinc, riboflavin, niacin, thiamin, vitamins B6 and B12, amino acids, and iron than white meat. Dark meats also contain more saturated fats, along with omega-3 and omega-6 fats." *(http://articles.mercola.com/sites/articles/archive/2007/11/01/what-s-the-difference-between-white-and-dark-meat.aspx)*

These differences do have a bearing on which is best for the various nutritional types. Protein types should eat dark meat, and carbo types should eat white meat. What should a mixed type eat? You guessed it– some of both.

One last warning about America's meat supply

We need to be super vigilant about a couple of other aspects of the meat industry—gas packaging, and brine injection systems. An article about these practices can be found in the pages of my very favorite magazine, "Mother Earth News."

(This magazine gives wonderful articles bi-monthly on how to live off the land, be sustainable, and honor this planet we live on.) The web address is *www.MotherEarthNews.com* and the article is titled "Shocking News About Meat." It is discomforting, indeed. To quote:

"Two of the biggest trends reshaping America's meat supply are *gas packaging* and *brine injection systems*. Manufacturers save millions of dollars in lost meat turnover with these technologies, which make meat appear fresh longer and pump "flavor" into factory-farmed meat, in the form of salt water and broth."

The article continues, "Finally, critics point out that saltwater pumping and gas packaging make it more likely that consumers will buy and eat spoiled meat, and almost certain that they'll be eating old meat without realizing it. Traditionally packaged ground beef has a shelf life of about five days, while modified atmospheric packaging can give ground beef a shelf life of 14 or even 28 days, says Tony Corbo of the Washington D.C.-based Food and Water Watch. In fact, *Consumer Reports* found in 2006 that three out of 10 gas-packed ground beef samples had spoiled by their use- or freeze-by date. But all of it still *looked* nice and red."

..."If you know what to look for, gas-packed meats are easy to recognize, although you have no way of knowing which gases are inside. The packages are stouter than the old familiar plastic-wrapped Styrofoam assembly, with a sealed clear plastic top that's often slightly puffed up by the gases trapped inside."

In summary, always buy organic meat, which uses vacuum packaging instead of gas packaging. If you have to buy case-ready meat conventionally packaged, always get one that has the plastic stuck to the meat. That way there is no gas involved.

Buying packaged cuts locally

For those who live in the Dawsonville or Ellijay, Georgia area, there is a wonderful farm called Mountain Valley Farm which is about 15 miles away from Amicalola Falls. They are USDA inspected and they sell grass-fed, grass-finished beef and heritage pork by the cut, frozen, as well as eggs and raw milk, the latter of which is technically for pet consumption only and is labeled as such.

Their information can be found at *www.LocalHarvest.org*. Once on the home page, in the search engine, enter "Mountain Valley Farm" and the zip code "30536" and you will be taken to their page. Click on "more" at the bottom and you'll see a beautiful picture of their farm and can get directions and contact information.

This is currently where I buy all of my meat because I live close to it. It is worth the drive, and lots of people even come up from Atlanta to purchase food there. I believe in supporting local farmers as much as possible and I encourage you to do so in your own area.

Low and Slow

Cooking the meat is the next thing to know how to do, now that you have decided that grass-fed beef is the best kind to purchase.

I know that one of the great American pastimes is grilling outdoors, but that is actually the worst way to prepare meat, because it creates advance glycation end-products (AGEs). As the name implies, AGEs contribute to premature aging, among other things. Cooking meat at low temperatures for longer periods (i.e., "Low and Slow") is the best way, as described in the following pages.

This next section is compliments of the American Grassfed Association, and will give you all of the information you need to ensure that your grass-fed beef cooks up tender and succulent. Please be sure to follow their advice, otherwise your beef will be tough and tasteless.

Tips for Cooking Grass-fed Beef

1. Your biggest culprit for tough grass fed beef is overcooking. This beef is made for rare to medium rare cooking. If you like well done beef, then cook your grass fed beef at very low temperatures in a sauce to add moisture.

2. Since grass fed beef is extremely low in fat, coat with virgin olive oil, truffle oil, or light oil for flavor enhancement and easy browning. The oil will also prevent drying and sticking.

3. We recommend marinating your beef before cooking especially lean cuts like NY Strip and Sirloin Steak. Choose a recipe that doesn't mask the delicate flavor of grass fed beef but enhances the moisture content. A favorite marinade using lemon, vinegar, wine, beer or bourbon is a great choice. If you choose to use bourbon, beer or vinegar, use slightly less than you would use for grain fed beef. Grass fed beef cooks quicker so the liquor or vinegar won't have as much time to cook off. For safe handling, always marinate in the refrigerator.

4. If you do not have time to marinate, just coat your thawed steak with your favorite rub, place on a solid surface, cover with plastic and pound your steak a few times to break down the connective tissue. As an added benefit your favorite rub will be pushed into your grass fed beef. Don't go overboard and flatten your beef unless your recipe calls for it. If you don't have a meat mallet, use a rolling pin or whatever you feel is safe and convenient.

5. Stove top cooking is great for any type of steak . . . including grass fed steak. You have more control over the temperature than on the grill. You can use butter in the final minutes when the heat is low to carry the taste of fresh garlic through the meat just like steak chefs.

6. Grass fed beef has high protein and low fat levels, so the beef will usually require 30% less cooking time and will continue to cook when removed from heat. For this reason, remove the beef from your heat source 10° before it reaches the desired temperature.

7. Use a thermometer to test for doneness and watch the thermometer carefully. Since grass fed beef cooks so quickly, your beef can go from perfectly cooked to over-cooked in less than a minute.

8. Let the beef sit covered and in a warm place for 8 to 10 minutes after removing from heat to let the juices redistribute.

9. Never use a fork to turn your beef . . . precious juices will be lost. Always use tongs.

10. Reduce the temperature of your grain fed beef recipes by 50° i.e. 275° for roasting or at the lowest heat setting in a crock pot. The cooking time will still be the same or slightly shorter even at the lower temperature. Again . . . watch your meat thermometer and don't overcook your meat. Use moisture from sauces to add to the tenderness when cooking your roast.

11. Never use a microwave to thaw your grass fed beef. Either thaw your beef in the refrigerator or for quick thawing place your vacuum sealed package in water for a few minutes.

12. Bring your grass fed meat to room temperature before cooking . . . do not cook it cold straight from a refrigerator.

13. Always pre-heat your oven, pan or grill before cooking grass fed beef.

14. When grilling, sear the meat quickly over a high heat on each side to seal in its natural juices and then reduce the heat to a medium or low to finish the cooking process. Also, baste to add moisture throughout the grilling process. Don't forget grass fed beef requires 30% less cooking time so watch your thermometer and don't leave your steaks unattended.

15. When roasting, sear the beef first to lock in the juices and then place in a pre-heated oven. Save your leftovers . . . roasted grass fed beef slices make great healthy luncheon meats with no additives or preservatives.

16. When preparing hamburgers on the grill, use caramelized onions, olives or roasted peppers to add low fat moisture to the meat while cooking. We add zero fat to our burgers (they are 85% to 90% lean) . . . so some moisture is needed to compensate for the lack of fat. Make sure you do not overcook your burgers . . . 30% less cooking time is required.

What I do is cook my ground beef in a frying pan on the stove, in some coconut oil. It is delicious and so healthy for you! I put it on medium low (electric stoves now are more efficient) and leave the inside pink so it doesn't take very long at all.

With this company, Whiteoak Pastures, I know that the meat has been handled well and therefore I have no qualms about eating it the way some people would term "raw." This meat is sold in all the states surrounding Georgia: Florida, Alabama, North Carolina, South Carolina, and Tennessee (and possibly some others).

The same is true for the beef I buy at Mountain Valley Farm, a local farm near me. If you ask around, you will eventually find a farm near you that sells this wonderful food.

Temperatures for cooking

The temperature that is used to cook meat makes a huge difference in its digestibility and nutrition in the body. Dr. Nancy Appleton has this to say about it:

"The higher the temperature that food is cooked, the longer it stays in the gut and the more difficult it becomes for our digestive mechanisms to digest it. This makes it more difficult for the food to absorb and function at a cellular level where it needs to work.

When the food can not function in the cells, the cells can become deficient and/or toxic which leads to deficiency and toxicity of the whole body making the body less able to function optimally...An immune response can be triggered by undigested food that gets into the bloodstream and must be treated as a foreign invader by the immune system." (*http://articles.mercola.com/sites/articles/archive/2002/05/29/over-cooking.aspx*) Please read the rest of the article to get a full understanding of this process.

Oven cooking

For anything cooked in the oven, the temperature should not go over 225°F. It should be cooked at 50% over the normal cooking time, or 150% of the original cooking time in total.

Therefore, say a chicken recipe that calls for cooking 1 hour at 350°F would need to be cooked for 1½ hours at 225°F. This keeps most of the nutrients available and is much healthier for you. Also, most stoves today are much more efficient and therefore you don't need to go over medium low in cooking meat.

Fish and To Eat Meat or Not

Fish, of course, is not technically meat, but I am including a discussion of it because it warrants mentioning. Fish would be a great source of nutrients but unfortunately, most of it is so contaminated with mercury that it is no longer a good choice.

My grandparents ran a hunting and fishing lodge in Sopchoppy, Florida for many years and my siblings and I grew up on the wonderful seafood found in the Gulf of Mexico area around there. I don't eat much from conventional sources anymore because it has been so contaminated.

And, of course, the problems with the BP Oil spill have only added to the existing contamination, so seafood is mostly off limits for me unless I can verify where it is caught.

If you catch fish from freshwater lakes and streams, they are most likely the safest you can get when fishing yourself. Be sure you are familiar with the headwaters and what is going into the water from upstream.

Dr. Mercola offers some more information to help you decide if you want to eat fish. "According to new U.S. Geological Survey study, scientists detected mercury contamination in every fish sampled in nearly 300 streams across the U.S.

About a quarter of these fish were found to contain mercury at levels exceeding the criterion for the protection of people who consume average amounts of fish, established by the U.S. Environmental Protection Agency. More than two-thirds of the fish exceeded the U.S. EPA level of concern for fish-eating mammals." *http://blogs.mercola.com/sites/vitalvotes/ archive/2009/09/15/new-evidence-on-mercury-in-fish.aspx*

To solve this problem I order my fish from the company Vital Choice (*www.vitalchoice.com*) because it has been third-party independently tested and shown to be the most free of mercury. These fish come from the pristine and pure waters off the coast of Alaska and are harvested in a sustainable manner.

Their salmon sausages are awesome, plus they are quick and easy to fix. Their canned tuna and salmon is the best I've ever tasted. Either makes a terrific salad. Just eating this fish once a week supplies you with Omega-3 benefits. You owe it to yourself to give it a try.

To eat or not to eat meat

One last subject to cover is whether or not to eat meat at all. Just as with conventional produce, you have to be aware of what's going on and choose your product accordingly.

Many vegetarians and vegans oppose eating meat on moral or ethical grounds, and I respect that. Unless I was starving, I don't think I could kill any animal. I'm very grateful that others are willing to do it for me.

Did you know that you kill the vegetables just as you do animals? Just because they can't scream and run away from you doesn't mean that they willingly want to be eaten.

Actually, they do scream in their own way. Read the book *The Secret Life of Plants* by Peter Tompkins and Christopher Bird for an eye opener. I planned on reading that book to bore me to sleep one night, but it was fascinating and I couldn't put it down.

There is also an article from the New York Times on how plants are sensitive to their environment and quickly react to it. They use many extraordinary tricks to fend off attackers and solicit help from afar. Go to *www.nytimes.com* and search for "Sorry Vegans: Brussels Sprouts Want To Live Too" by Natalie Angier.

I personally tried vegetarianism and found that it didn't work for me. I was constantly hungry and the wheat didn't agree with me (I later found out I am gluten sensitive). So, I had to give it up. Plus, I gained weight and was tired most of the time.

For me, I have thrived on the mixed nutritional type diet with small amounts of good, organic meat. I don't want to eat meat from animals who have been treated inhumanely, but I go out of my way and spend extra money to get good-for-me kinds of meat.

I have endeavored to give alternatives that take vegans and vegetarians into account and all of my meatless recipes will work well for them. My sincere hope is that there will be something here for everyone.

The Incredible Egg

Eggs are a wonderful source of high quality protein and fat in an easily transported package. You can hard boil them, and take them with you on airplanes to eat instead of being forced to eat airline food. They beat the high prices of hotel food, too!

The best way to eat eggs, according to Dr. Mercola, is raw. Now I know that might gross some of you out, but bear with me as I explain. Cooking eggs, as with most things, destroys vital nutrients, which remain intact when you consume them raw.

I put a raw egg into my Morning Wake-up Shake each day and you cannot tell that it is in there. Egg yolks have very fragile proteins, so you don't want to beat them in. With a variable speed blender (like a Vitamix), turn it on just barely enough to get the egg to go to the bottom of the blender, and then immediately turn it off.

If you are a protein type or a mixed nutritional type, eggs are a perfect food for your metabolism. Raw is best, and scrambled is the worst way to eat them, since egg protein is easily damaged on a molecular level by being beaten.

Important raw egg guidelines

To eat eggs raw, there are some guidelines that you need to follow. If you buy them free-range, from a local farmer, you will be amazed at how good they are. I am fortunate to have found just such a place—a family in which their two oldest boys raise the chickens as their business.

The boys are home-schooled so the chickens get to run around in the yard all day and eat what chickens are supposed to eat–bugs! It might come as a surprise to many of you, but chickens are not vegetarians and they receive valuable protein from the insects they eat.

As such, they also provide organic pest control in the garden. Their manure, since it is in small quantities, adds organic matter to the soil and thus enriches the garden as well.

For what I will be explaining next, you can go to my website to see pictures of each of the parts. That will help you to better understand what I am talking about. The address is *www.HealthyEatingOnTheRun.com/egg-nutrition.html.*

Free range eggs

In commercial egg production, the designation "Free Range" can be used if the chickens raised in warehouse-like chicken houses have an open door at some point during the day. They don't necessarily have to go out the door, and usually don't. As opposed to that environment, I buy eggs from happy chickens that wander around in chicken yards. Their eggs are different.

First off, their shells are much harder than conventional eggs, and you almost have to whack them against something to get them to break. Secondly, once you get them to break, the yolks are a really bright orange-yellow instead of the pale yellow you get from the store. They are usually bigger, too, sometimes even having double yolks.

The other neat thing is that you don't have to refrigerate truly free range eggs if you don't wash them until you are ready to use them. I get mine straight from the hen's nests (or sometimes the ground), and store them on my kitchen counter in a cute little wire container. They have mud and hay stuck on them quite often. (See picture on my website.)

My eggs keep on the counter for up to four weeks. When you think about it, most of the world does not refrigerate their eggs and they do just fine.

According to Julie, my egg lady and the mother of the two egg entrepreneurs, there is a membrane on the egg, called the bloom, that stays intact until you wash it. If they have been washed, they need to be refrigerated. Once refrigerated, they need to be kept cold until used.

The safety of raw eggs

Because of the slight risk of salmonella infection, you do have to take some precautions before using free range eggs. Please test them to make sure they are okay to use. Dr. Mercola estimated that the risk of contracting an infection from eggs is one in 30,000. That is for store bought eggs. The risk from free-range eggs is even smaller. *(http://articles.mercola.com/sites/articles/archive/2002/11/13/eggs-part-two.aspx)*

Always practice good hygiene. Wash your hands thoroughly after handling free-range eggs. Julie's next door neighbor contracted salmonella after gathering her own eggs from her own chickens, then sitting down to eat lunch without washing her hands.

Once you have washed the egg you plan to use in your smoothie or in other recipes, you need to test it to see if it's good. This is done very simply.

How to test eggs for safety

Take a glass or jar and put *cold* water in it (not lukewarm), and add a bit of salt. Don't waste your good salt on this–just buy and use a cheap kind. Then take the egg to be tested and drop it (carefully!) into your salt water. (You can use tongs to do this if you prefer.)

If tiny bubbles come out of the egg in a stream, the outer shell has been compromised and the egg should be discarded. That has only happened to me once in two years, and that was with store-bought eggs.

A fresh egg will sink directly to the bottom and lie on its side. If it bobs a little bit before lying on the bottom, it is about one week old. If it stands up on the bottom, pointed end down, it is probably about three weeks old and is still perfectly good to eat.

If it floats half way up, use it immediately, as it won't be good for long. Caution: if it floats on top of the water, throw it away and don't even think about eating it.

Testing an egg in this way works because eggs lose both moisture and carbon dioxide as they age, and that makes them more buoyant.

Second test for safety

There is a second test that you need to do on your eggs, and that is to ALWAYS break them into a separate dish or ramekin first before adding them to other ingredients. An egg could do fine on the floating test and still be bad inside.

This happened to me once with a very big egg that I figured was a double yolk. Sure enough, it was, and when I cracked it open into my recipe mixture, one yolk was fine and the other was black as the Ace of Spades. That was my last egg, so I had to throw the whole thing out and start over. Thus the need to break an egg into a SEPARATE dish before adding to your recipe! You'll be happy you did.

Of course, it goes without saying that if you open an egg and it is discolored or smells bad, discard it immediately. You'll know at once. (They don't call it the "rotten egg smell" for nothing!) After you develop the habit of testing your fresh eggs, you can feel secure in enjoying one of nature's perfect foods any time you want.

Recycling egg shells

There is one other thing I want to mention here. I recycle or compost everything that I can and the eggshells go in to my back door composter. Because I am blessed to live across the valley from Amicalola Falls, one of Georgia's most beautiful state parks, we do have a problem with bears.

I have to wash all of my eggshells before they go into the composter in order to keep bears away from them. It's best to do that anyway to keep other critters from causing trouble.

Chapter 5

Growing Your Own Food

The best way to ensure that you eat healthy food is to grow it yourself. Then you can be sure of what kind of soil and pest control (hopefully natural) you use.

This is easier than you may realize if you think outside the box, or in some cases, inside a box. If you have any sunny space at all, be it patio or deck, you can grow things. And if you don't, you can still grow things hydroponically. Where there's a will, there's a way.

I have a fairly large deck on the back of my house and I use Earth boxes, big pots, and Topsy Turvy planters to grow my food. It is, unfortunately, facing North, but during the long days of summer I can grow quite a lot.

The Earth boxes have their own nutrient and watering system and you can't overwater them at all. Any excess water just goes right on through and out the overflow opening. You do have to keep them watered regularly, especially in times of drought (I add water every two days when it doesn't rain). Even though I have Earth boxes, I think the ones from "A Garden Patch" are a better value. (*www.aGardenPatch.com*)

I have grown garlic, bell peppers, yellow squash, zucchini squash, strawberries, blueberries, broccoli, chard, cantaloupes, Stevia, and tomatoes with varying degrees of success. I don't use regular growing spaces for two reasons.

First, the soil here is beyond lousy. We have nothing but Georgia red clay here (as in "Gone With the Wind") and it won't grow anything, even with attempts at amending it. That's why I gave up and now use raised beds and containers.

Second, we have problems with bears and other critters. We love our mountain home, but it IS two miles from a state park, where bears roam freely. Therefore, we have to keep our bird feeders and produce up off of the ground in order to keep them away from the food. We also have tons of deer, rabbits, and other critters who would love to share our bounty.

So up on the deck it goes, and the system has worked very well. At the present time, no bears have tried to climb up the deck supports, although they are quite capable of it.

74

Using pots and planters means that you can control the soil, and the nutrients that go in it. I put my Earth boxes up on concrete blocks in order to make it easier on my back, both to water them and to harvest produce. Water can run out more easily as well, which is a plus.

I am a new gardener with not much experience, so every year is a new challenge and experiment. I lost all of my broccoli and squash the summer of 2009, but other things did well so overall, I am pleased with the results.

Aerogardens

If you don't have the outdoor space (or just don't want to deal with bugs or other problems of growing things outside), you can always use Aerogardens. I've had mine for a number of years and just love them. Nothing beats fresh cherry tomatoes in January!

They come with planting kits that are guaranteed to grow. All you do is put the seed kits in the holes, add water and the nutrients that they provide, and watch stuff grow!

Okay, so maybe that isn't *all* you have to do. You do have to check the water, especially when herbs are growing, and keep it topped off. You'll sometimes hear when the water is low because the base makes a gurgling sound, so you know it's time to add some water. You also add more nutrients every two weeks when the lights flash, and raise the lights up when the plants grow tall. The system tells you what to do-it's pretty minimal, and easy.

When the plants start growing, you have to trim them back (you can eat the trimmings, usually). Also, make sure any dead leaves, etc., are cleared out, the same as if you were gardening outside. The reward is fresh food, even in the dead of winter, a fair trade off in my opinion. The plant kits include salad greens, bell peppers, tomatoes, various herbs, green beans, romaine lettuce, and flowers, if you don't want to grow food.

You can find pictures of the Aerogardens on my website. Here is an address that will take you directly to more information: *www.HealthyEatingOnTheRun.com/grow-foods.html.*

I'm not too pleased with the latest Topsy Turvey planters that I bought. They fell apart after just one year of use. The ones that I had bought previously lasted many years, so they must have changed the composition of the plastic. I don't know that I would try them again without more research on how well they will hold up.

"Gardeners Supply" offers an upside down planter that is much more sturdy, and I'm sure there are other brands out there. You can even make your own. Instructions abound on the Internet.

For the 2011 growing season, I have switched to Square Foot Gardening. Brian made 4'x4' square boxes on raised legs for me so that they are waist high. We put them in the front yard instead of the back, because that is the only place that gets any sun. So far they have been doing fairly well, and the boxes are durable and will last for many years.

There are all kinds of options for someone willing to buy a book or two to learn new things or to search the internet for information. I took a Master Gardening class at the beginning of this year (2011), and have lots of book learning. Now I just need to implement it and get more hands-on experience under my belt. I encourage you to do the same.

Growing Stevia

With just a little bit of effort, you can grow your own sweetener and harvest it yearly for yourself and your family. Since a little bit of it goes a long way, you don't need much to supply your sweetener needs for a whole year.

I found organic seeds for Stevia at Whole Foods market, and after I had already bought those, I accidentally discovered that they sold the whole plant as well. The plants over-wintered very well indoors and came back again from the root the next spring.

In the year 2009, one branch of my Stevia decided it liked my tomatoes and reached over to their pot. It then proceeded to plant itself into the soil there, so now I have two Stevia plants instead of one. I just transplanted the new one into something smaller and brought them both inside to wait for warm weather again.

You should harvest the leaves before the plants start to flower, which in Georgia would be about mid-September. If you start to see flowers, pinch them off and then harvest the leaves as soon as possible. By harvesting, I mean just pull the leaves off of the plant and wash them if they have dirt on them. Then set them out to dry on a piece of paper towel until no longer moist. After that, you can put them in an open flat dish and let them dry until crumbly.

Once completely dry, you can run them through a coffee grinder (clean, of course) until finely chopped or to a powder consistency, and then store them in an airtight container. You will need to experiment to see how much to use, as sweetness can vary. If you wait until many flowers have formed, the Stevia will start to have a bitter aftertaste, so harvest them before that happens. (I found this out the hard way!)

To use the leaves, put a few in a fine strainer and hold it over your cup. Pour hot water through the leaves to sweeten your beverage. You'll have to experiment with the quantity of leaves you use to adjust the sweetness. You can use the powder directly in your cup.

Types of Stevia

Stevia comes in many forms, from powder, to extract, to whole leaves, to liquid. I prefer the Stevia extract from "NOW" brand and know how much to use because I am familiar with it. Remember, you can always add more, but you can't take it out if you've put in too much. Extract, as opposed to powder, does not have the aftertaste that some people find to be objectionable.

As stated earlier, Stevia is 200-300 times sweeter than sugar, so use it sparingly. "NOW" brand includes a very small spoon to use as a serving. To see what it looks like, go to my website *www.HealthyEatingOnTheRun.com/growing-stevia.html* for a picture of it. There is a regular teaspoon beside the "NOW" spoon to illustrate how really small it is.

Some people think that Stevia has a bitter aftertaste, so try different brands to see what works best for you. Don't give up if you do try one brand and don't like it. It does have a slightly anise or licorice flavor to it naturally, some brands more so than others.

Brands of Stevia

"NOW" brand has a wonderful French Vanilla flavor Stevia in packets. Since so little is needed, to have a quantity that looked familiar, there had to be a lot of filler added to it. I'm leery of this, as I found that I liked this particular variety of Stevia a bit too much.

It says that it has "natural flavorings" in it and that it does contain milk, so it might have dried milk added to it. Please see the "All About Milk" section (page 40) to read about the dangers involved in that. It could also have had sugar in the form of dextrose in it, which is what the artificial sweeteners do, and they are not required to put that on the label.

I called the company to find out exactly what constituted "natural flavorings" and was told that it was proprietary information. They couldn't give it out because their competitors might copy it. They did say that I could ask for specific things and they could tell me if it was in the product or not.

I asked about MSG, and they said "No, it is not included." But I didn't ask if it had MSG under any of the other names it goes by. Something in the packets made me almost addicted, and I consumed way too much. I considered that to be a clue and gave up the French Vanilla flavor, although I do still use "NOW" brand Stevia extract.

Luo Han Guo sweetener

I had to learn to switch back and forth between Stevia and Luo Han Guo as sweeteners because I developed a slight sensitivity to the Stevia. I wonder now if it wasn't some other ingredient in the French Vanilla that was causing the problem.

My theory is, the simpler and more natural the product is, the better it is for you. There is less likelihood of having any adverse reaction if it is just one, made-by-nature substance.

Recycling

Recycling is one of the things that is near and dear to my heart. What is the importance of recycling? Well, if we don't start taking care of this planet we live on, it won't be worth living on anymore.

That's one reason I like the Grab and Go system so much—there is no waste to throw away. The United States has a huge problem with its garbage.

This is also a global problem. Check out the following website. *http://www.mindfully.org/ Plastic/Ocean/Moore-Trashed-PacificNov03.htm.* This page describes a garbage patch of plastic debris that is the size of the state of Texas! The area is devoid of any sea life, because it can't be sustained.

Fortunately, I see signs that this situation is changing, and I'm greatly heartened by that. "Reduce, Reuse, Recycle" is coming back into vogue. There is a rising movement towards uncluttering lives and going by the motto "live simply, that others may simply live."

Frugality is coming back with the slogan "Use it up, wear it out, make it do, or do without." The bad economy has had a lot to do with it, of course, but I say it's about time!

My town of Dawsonville has a well-used and important recycling program with a dumpster that is under a shelter so that you can bring recyclables even in the rain. You don't have to divide things up anymore, either, which makes it easier, too. They somehow separate things out later with fans, magnets, and other systems. Some companies separate by hand, also.

Our program accepts office paper, newspaper, junk mail (even with inserts), magazines, phone books, glass bottles and jars (all colors), plastic items numbered 1-7 (check the bottom for the number), aluminum beverage cans and steel/tin ones, and chipboard, which is cereal type boxes (with the plastic liner removed) and cardboard, flattened where possible. You shouldn't have significant food residues on any item you recycle. For example, pizza boxes are not acceptable.

For a very informative article on what happens to these items through the recycling process, please go to this site: *http://www.wholeliving.com/article/sorting-it-out*. Recycling is so important because it really does help the environment in many ways.

An excellent guide to healthier food uses of plastics with a Smart Plastics Guide can be found at *http://www.healthobservatory.org/library.cfm?RefID=77083*. This tells you what each of those numbers (1-7) mean and how each one can affect your health and that of your family.

It details the dangers of Bisphenol A (BPA) and DEHA, two components of plastic, and what they can do to your body. In addition, it offers tips for avoiding these and tells you how to use plastic safely.

One of the important recycling advantages is that you don't have as much trash to put out. For most people, it's no big deal, but if you live out in the boondocks like I do, it makes a huge difference.

We have to take our garbage to the dump and pay 50¢ per bag for it. Because I recycle, it takes me at least four to six weeks to gather enough household garbage to fill up an entire bag. I don't buy things with a lot of packaging, either, and I take reusable bags in with me when I go shopping. That saves me money and makes life simpler, indeed.

Recycling idea

Here's a nifty idea that will save you a lot of money versus mail-order catalog varieties. I save my baggies and zip lock plastic sandwich bags and reuse them. I wash them out and then put them over my homemade drying rack to dry out. Just be sure to wash them out really well, the same way you would a plate, mug or dish.

I took an old toothbrush holder and put chopsticks in it to hold the bags to dry. Pencils would work just as well if you don't have any chopsticks. You can go to my website at *www.HealthyEatingOnTheRun.com/recycling.html* to see a picture of it.

If you have a toothbrush holder to use, by all means go ahead and use it. I have one that has a bottom, but the lid detaches for easy cleaning. It works very well. If you use a holder with an open base, water will go everywhere, plus it may be unstable since it is lighter. When buying a new holder, look for these features.

A heavier holder won't tip over as easily, and you'll be glad it is easy to reach inside to clean. Ceramic is more stable, but probably won't have a top that comes off.

Composting

Another aspect of recycling is composting, and if you grow anything at all, this is something that would be beneficial for you to do. Not only does it keep things out of landfills (where it creates methane gas), it also helps to enrich your soil so that you get better nutrition out of what you grow and eat.

You can start out as simply as piling up kitchen scraps in a corner of your yard, but optimally, you should turn the pile to distribute the heat better. It could also attract rodents and other critters and rain will wash some of the nutrients into the ground. But it's simple and easy to do and I highly recommend that you try it.

A better way is to buy a compost tumbler. I tried the large garden one but did not have any luck with it. The lady at the company tried so hard to help me with it, giving me extra time and extra accessories, but it just didn't work. She said that was only the second time in her 20 year career there that she couldn't help someone be successful with it.

I sent that one back (a major feat in itself) and got the "Back Porch ComposTumbler" instead. With it, I had major success and it is super easy. It's almost like a bottomless pit where I can constantly throw in scraps and once a year take out the finished compost.

Here's a list of what can go into a compost pile:

Vegetable scraps, kitchen scraps, fruit scraps, used paper towels if no chemicals are on them, egg shells, leaves, grass clippings, plant prunings, dead flowers, straw or hay, coffee grounds, and tea bags. If any items are large, cutting them into smaller pieces will make it easier to decompose. Citrus peels will need to be cut into small pieces because they take a long time to break down otherwise.

Do not compost meat, bones, fatty substances (like cheese) or fish scraps (they will attract pests), perennial weeds (they can be spread with the compost) or diseased plants. Do not include pet manure in compost that will be used on food crops.

Banana peels, peach peels and orange rinds may contain pesticide residue, and should be kept out of the compost. Black walnut leaves should not be composted. Sawdust may be added to the compost, but should be mixed or scattered thinly to avoid clumping. Be sure sawdust is clean, with no machine oil or chain oil residues from cutting equipment.

With the "Back Porch ComposTumbler" you can compost during the winter, or at lease keep adding things in. They won't actually decompose until the weather warms up some. However, the microbes are what cause it to decompose, so the weather does not affect it the process that much.

You don't have to worry about the ratio of nitrogen (green things) to carbon (brown things) with it, either. If it starts to smell like ammonia, just add some brown leaves in to balance it.

Another thing you won't need is a compost pail to keep in your kitchen to hold scraps until you have enough to take outside. My fancy-schmancy compost pail is a quart-size yogurt container. When the container gets too yucky, I just rinse it out, recycle it, and start with a clean one.

Here's another good tip. If you have those pesky fruit flies in your kitchen, here's a way to get rid of them. Just put a large zip lock type plastic bag over the yogurt container with the side of it hanging over the kitchen counter a bit. (See my website for a picture of my trap.)

They will fly under the edge of the bag into the container and you can just pull the edges of the bag together to trap them and take them outside. Put the scraps into the composter and shake the bag to release the fruit flies. Simple and easy and you save yourself a lot of money over buying the catalog items to take care of both problems.

An alternate method is to put a little apple cider vinegar in the bottom of a jar, and put a drop of dish soap in it to break the surface tension. Then form a cone from a piece of paper (or use a #4 coffee filter). Make sure there is a small hole for the fruit flies to enter the jar. They will become trapped when they can't find the hole again to fly out. Simply take the trap and dump it when you are ready to start over.

Composting made a huge difference in both my flower gardens and my vegetable gardens. In my opinion, it is well worth taking the time to recycle kitchen scraps into "black gold" for your yard.

E-cycling

If you have e-waste (electronics) to get rid of, be sure to check out *www.earth911.com* or *www.ecyclingcentral.com* to see what companies in your area might take them. Please don't just trash them as they contain many toxic substances that will contaminate groundwater and the environment.

Once or twice a year, my local community has an e-cycling day where they will take electronics to be recycled. Watch your newspaper for a possible one in your area.

Chapter 6

My Journey to Wellness

I have been on my journey to wellness basically all of my life, but my real turning point came in the year 2000 when I finally moved up to the North Georgia mountains, where I reside today. I am blessed to live right across the valley from Amicalola Falls, one of our beautiful state parks, with my partner Brian Fraser. We have a beautiful view of the falls in our backyard.

I built a real log home with six-inch thick log walls for the outside of the house. The plumber/electrician I hired was supposed to be retired, but he took on work if he liked the job. He worked for time plus materials, and said if I wanted to cut down on costs, he would show me how to do the work and I could help him.

I took him up on his offer, and learned more than I ever wanted to know about how houses are built, but it was a great education and has served me well in the interim years. I dug the ditches for the plumbing and pulled electrical wires until I thought my hands would fall off. But I absolutely adore my house and where I live now.

Brian had bought the lot next to me with his then wife Donna. They eventually divorced. She kept the thriving massage practice that they had both built up in Stone Mountain and gave him the land with a mortgage and a little log cabin storage shed on it. He told me he was just going to stay in the shed and take showers over at the State Park with the park pass he had purchased.

The more I thought about that, the more unfair it seemed, so I offered to let him stay in the little apartment I had built downstairs in my house in case I ever needed to bring my elderly father here to live with me (I did but that's a different story).

He could stay for free in return for helping me finish my house. Like most people, I had run out of money in building it. He had been a master carpenter for 27 years before becoming a massage therapist so it was a good deal for me, too.

Job changes

When I moved to the mountains, I had been doing healing work (Reiki and ear candling) in Atlanta and I expected to just keep my clients and go back to Atlanta as needed. For some reason, probably because I detested driving in Atlanta traffic, that just dried up. Brian also was going to Atlanta to do massage work.

I checked with a local resort up here to see if they needed a massage therapist and it turns out they did. So he started working there in March of 2003.

I kept trying to find local work and finally gave up. I told Brian, "Teach me how to do massage" and he did. So now we both run the Spa at this resort and he is my life partner as well as my business partner. It worked out well for both of us until I started having problems with my hands.

Raw foods enter the picture

In the year 2000, before I left Atlanta, I took a course in raw foods from Brenda Cobb at the Living Foods Institute. Later, I also took classes from Jackie and Gideon Graff at Sprout Raw Foods and these people, along with Bruce Fife for the coconut flour baked goods, have been the inspiration for my recipes. I owe them a huge thanks for all their teachings.

That was the beginning of my journey to wellness in earnest. I felt that the raw food diet was the one for me, and I actually gave away all of my other cookbooks. I ate only the raw foods but found that I was gaining weight and was tired all the time. So I was really puzzled because, intuitively, the raw food felt good for me.

I started adding in some meat and cheese and then the brain fog lifted and the tiredness went away somewhat. I kept exploring and searching on the internet and finally ran across Dr. Mercola's site. His three different nutritional types really made sense to me and after finding out which type I was (mixed type), I stuck strictly to the rules for my type and started feeling much better.

In 2006, two of the owners of the resort where I worked, started talking about having a Wellness Center and I was really excited about that. We went forward with the plans for it and in 2008, moved the Spa from its first location underneath the office, to its present location at the house that was the residence of the patriarch who first started the resort.

It was named Anidawehi Spa and Wellness Center, in honor of the Cherokee Native Americans who first lived on the land. The move was very stressful, because we were still trying to do massages while doing much of the renovation work ourselves, especially Brian.

At that time I was also trying to get the information together to teach classes on raw and alternative foods, to help others find optimal health. It was overwhelming to say the least, the same as the website has been, and the book, but I persevered. The end result was I burned out my adrenal glands to insufficiency, almost to the point of adrenal failure.

The cause of the burnout

What precipitated all of this was multifaceted. I had to move my Dad from Albuquerque, New Mexico to Georgia when my beloved step-mom died in 2004. We drove his belongings to my house and he stayed with us for a month while I searched for an assisted living home for him. We live on the side of a mountain on ten acres, and it wasn't safe for him to be here because he had Sundowner's as well as Alzheimer's and would wander if left alone.

In 2005, a law was passed requiring massage therapists to be licensed. So, I also went to massage school while still working full time. Halfway through school I found out I could have been grandfathered in and didn't need the schooling. However, I decided to go ahead and finish, anyway, so there could be no questions later.

I was in charge of Daddy's care in an assisted living home for 4½ years, until he died from Alzheimer's in 2008. Someone once said that disease is the long goodbye and they were absolutely right. It was devastating for me and took a huge toll on my health.

Then I had to settle Daddy's estate, which took an entire year after his death, and pay all the taxes, etc. Any one of these things by itself I could have handled okay, but with all of them together I was simply overwhelmed. I have finally come to realize that I am not Superwoman and I can't do it all, but it was an expensive lesson.

The adrenal fatigue then negatively impacted my thyroid, which caused a chain reaction with my female hormones, making menopausal symptoms almost unbearable. I was having hot flashes every two hours, day and night, and the night ones woke me up each time to throw the covers off for a minute and then pull them back once it was over. I was so sleep deprived, I would fly off the handle at anything and everything, and was even having mild anxiety attacks.

Since everything in the body is related, everything combined made my thyroid condition even worse. It enlarged, to try to process more iodine. On ultrasound, there was a growth that showed "some vascularity." A subsequent biopsy showed "atypical" cells. Three doctors recommended surgical removal of my thyroid, but I said "No."

I believe strongly in holistic alternative medicine and I was not going undergo thyroid removal until I had tried everything possible to see if the growth could be reduced on its own. That was in 2009, and I started pursuing my journey to wellness in earnest.

I'm going to a place in Atlanta now called Progressive Medical Center and I am finally getting well. I'm on bioidentical hormones compounded specifically for my body, and they have been a Godsend. All of the menopausal symptoms have gone away and I can finally sleep at night with no hot flashes.

I'm even nice to be around now and don't fly off the handle (much) anymore. We're still trying to get the rest of my body balanced out but I'm feeling significantly better, and I'm back on track again!

Other issues show up

The other thing was that I was packing on pounds around my middle in spite of rigorous diet and exercise, and the numbers on my triglycerides, cholesterol and fasting blood sugar levels all kept creeping up. I had no energy, and exercise was horrendously difficult to do. I knew something was definitely wrong but my TSH (thyroid stimulating hormone) tests showed up normal.

It was only after I went to a holistic doctor that he said my thyroid was malfunctioning. He did a test for free T-3 and T-4 and found out I wasn't utilizing them properly at all. So even if I was producing enough thyroid hormones, my body wasn't using them effectively. Dr. Mercola says that if your TSH score is over 1.5 on a scale of .03 to 3, you are hypothyroid. My score was 1.7 and I was severely hypothyroid, with all the symptoms.

My naturopathic doctor had put me on a strict regimen of Iodoral tablets and Armour thyroid pills, with a thyroid cream to administer nightly. Finally it began to take effect. As of March of 2010, I had dropped 30 pounds of excess weight that was all around my middle. Excess abdominal weight is one symptom of thyroid problems.

I also found out that it didn't matter what foods I ate or didn't eat, or how much I exercised. As long as the thyroid was out of kilter, that fat was going to stay there because it was storing excess iodine for my body to use.

I couldn't take the time to listen to my body until after my Dad passed away, but my symptoms were trying to tell me that something was terribly wrong with my body. Daddy died in April, 2008 and in December of that year, I went to my first doctor.

As long as the adrenals are not functioning well, you are not going to be making enough cortisol, either. While that might seem like a good thing, it is not. Your body needs cortisol to function, especially for exercise. I used to walk three miles a day, five days a week religiously, no matter what the weather was like.

I found out that I was doing my body a grave disservice by forcing myself to exercise, thinking I was doing the right thing. It takes cortisol to exercise and you use it up when you do. If you don't have enough, it will put you flat on your back if you keep pushing your body. This I discovered the hard way.

My legs felt like lead weights when I tried to go up the steps to the road where I walk, and I was absolutely exhausted afterwards. I could only do it late in the day because there were many times I had to go lie down and rest afterwards.

There was definitely no "runner's high" of euphoria for me anymore. My body felt tired, as if I had not slept enough for weeks in a row, with a sort of borderline sick-to-my-stomach feeling. I simply had to quit exercising–I couldn't do it anymore.

Like many people, I have fought a weight problem pretty much all of my life. I even tried liposuction one time in a desperate attempt to get the fat off of me. I saw 500 cc of fat go literally down a tube and thought that was the answer. It all came back within a month.

I truly believe that I have had thyroid and adrenal problems most of my life. My poor body was just trying to take care of me and I didn't understand that. I need to honor and appreciate it more for its innate wisdom.

I know now that I am on the right path on my journey to wellness. I feel better when I eat the raw vegetables but I also know that I need good organic meat and raw cheese as well for my optimum health.

Hypothyroidism is on the rise

Subclinical hypothyroidism is epidemic in this country and people keep being told that it is all in their heads. We are NOT getting enough iodine here in the U.S. for a multitude of reasons, and we need to change that.

That is one of the reasons that I did this book and my website, to raise awareness of the problem. So many of us, women especially, are being told "It's all in your head," when we complain of symptoms to our doctors.

Background Information

The average person goes to ten different doctors before one finally tries something new and finds the problem. Most just look at TSH scores and say "You're fine." Well, if I'm so fine, why do I feel this way? You just have to keep digging until someone listens to you.

This next section on Thyroid Disease goes into much more detail. If you suspect you have a problem with either hypo- or hyperthyroidism, please check out the resources on this page. Perhaps you'll be on a journey to wellness soon, too.

If you would like to see before and after pictures of me along the way, you can go to my website at *www.HealthyEatingOnTheRun.com/my-journey-to-wellness.html*. I had the classic beer belly and I don't drink liquor or beer. In fact, I can't stand either one.

I have also decided to go all natural and have quit coloring my hair. I decided I liked the "highlights" that are in my hair now—I've earned every one of them!

[The following is taken from my website, and illustrates my progress in this journey.]

Health Update

May 27, 2010.

I just had another ultrasound done last week and I got the results back on Monday of this week. The growth on my thyroid had been 2.9 cm and it is now 2.3 cm. It is going down!

Naturopathy takes longer to work but it lets the body do its own healing. I went back to my wonderful Dr. Burdette yesterday and we are tweaking the supplements I am taking and adding more adrenal support.

I have dropped another three pounds and I fully expect to have my thyroid totally back to normal functioning. I feel very blessed.

June 22, 2010

My latest tests show that my adrenals are back to working normally now so I am delighted. I'm going to try to get back into walking again if it will ever cool down enough.

That may have to wait until September because I don't want to stress myself out again. We're still cutting down on supplements but until my thyroid is back to normal, I'm still on some meds. Happy days are here again!

February 17, 2011

I have now dropped down to 130 pounds on a 5'9" frame without even trying. That's 43 pounds off and I still haven't gotten back on an exercise program yet. I've had to go out and buy new clothes, which are a size 8! I'm so thrilled!

That tells me that all of the weight gain was purely thyroid, and the way I have been eating is perfect for my health. I still would like to get my waist measurement down from 32" but if it never happens, I'll be satisfied.

Thyroid Disease

This page has more in depth information on thyroid disease, the causes and cures. The article on Dr. Mercola's website described some of my symptoms exactly. If you even suspect that you may be experiencing issues with your thyroid, please take the time to read it. *http://articles.mercola.com/sites/articles/archive/2009/02/21/fatigue-dry-skin-gaining-weight-see-why-youd-better-check-your-thyroid-.aspx.*

The symptoms that I had included weight gain around my middle, in spite of eating healthy and exercising regularly, and very dry skin, so much so that the heels of my feet were actually cracking open.

I also had fatigue so bad that I would literally fall over asleep in my chair while sitting at my computer. There were times when I just had to have a nap in the afternoon, and I was not refreshed when I woke up.

All of the hair on my body fell out, too. It was nice not to have to shave my underarms and legs, but the hair on my head started to thin out as well. The body hair is back now but my head hair is still on the thin side. That is slowly changing for the better.

During the time I was so sick, I did not ever have constipation because of the raw food that I ate, and I had four to five bowel movements a day, which is the norm for me. I was not sensitive to cold, but my hands and feet always felt cold to the touch. Probably the hot flashes negated the sensation of coldness so I wasn't really aware of it.

These are the main symptoms of thyroid problems, so if you have any of these, be sure to see your doctor and have them test more than TSH. You will probably have to go to an alternative medicine or naturopathic doctor to get that done properly.

The Weston A. Price Foundation has sponsored seminars, and released a series of DVDs, all dealing with the subject of thyroid disorders. I ordered all of the DVDs from these sessions and they were very helpful to me.

Thyroid and iodine information

The following information is summarized from various sources on the WAP website. The WAPF Wise Traditions conference had a whole series of lectures on iodine deficiency. Contrary to popular belief, low iodine is widespread in America. It causes all sorts of health problems, including thyroid disease, cancer, and Down's Syndrome.

The reasons we are deficient include the fact that most of us don't consume enough iodine, and that we consume many substances which block iodine absorption in our body. There are halogens in our water including fluoride, chlorine, and perchlorate (rocket fuel).

Goitrogens, which also block iodine uptake, are widely distributed in our food supply. One is bromide, which is in most commercial bread, as well as some soft drinks (Mountain Dew for example). Probably the biggest single goitrogen we ingest is soy, which is everywhere.

Soybean oil is in salad dressing, mayonnaise, commercial baby formula, and almost all packaged cakes, candies chips, and crackers. Almost all restaurants cook their food in soybean oil. To make matters worse, most of the cows, poultry and pigs in this country are fed a diet of industrial corn and soybeans. It can creep into our diets in insidious ways.

One of the WAPF seminar speakers was Dr. David Brownstein, a Board-Certified Family Physician and author of eight books on healthy diets, iodine and thyroid issues, and natural healing. Notes from his lecture are provided below:

- We are all toxic with bromide, and it is a waste of money to even test for it

- The thyroid gland develops in the first trimester in the fetus

- If you are deficient in iodine, you will have increased risk of spontaneous abortion, or premature birth

- Iodine deficiency can lead to ovarian cysts, cysts in breasts, infertility, and menstrual disorders

- Iodine deficiency can lead to increased risk of Alzheimer's disease

- Iodine can help get people off insulin and diabetes medication

- 47% of breastfeeding women are iodine deficient in their milk

- Iodine deficiency increases ADD, ADHD, and decreases IQ

- We need iodine to be able to use cholesterol correctly in the body

- Iodine is necessary for the production of ALL hormones

- All cysts are an iodine deficiency, which if left untreated WILL turn into nodules, then fibroids, then cancer

- The longer seaweed is out of the water from where it originated, the less iodine will be in it; it will dissipate out in a gaseous form

- Iodine is antibacterial, anti-parasitic, anti-fungal, anti-cancer, and is a detox agent

- You need a combination of BOTH iodine and iodide to be effective

- More iodine is needed during puberty as the breasts are growing

- Only 10% of the iodine in iodized salt is bio-available

- Most pesticides/insecticides contain bromide, fluoride, and chlorine

- Bromide has no known role in the body, and it is a goitrogen

- People with cancer need very large doses of iodine

Another seminar speaker was Dr. Janet Lang, BA, DC. She has been in practice for 28 years, and among her many credits, she was a contributing author of *The Heart of the Healer*. She now consults, researches, and teaches Functional Endocrinology seminars across the country.

- It is important to fix the adrenals FIRST, before the thyroid. If you are having thyroid symptoms, you have already exhausted your adrenals. The thyroid will not respond until you treat the adrenals.

- The thyroid is the largest of all seven endocrine glands

- If the thyroid has sufficient iodine, it exerts a profound anti-microbial and antiseptic effect body wide

- All hormones are made from cholesterol, CHOLESTEROL is GOOD!

- Estrogen dominance can produce the same type of symptoms as thyroid imbalance, though there is nothing wrong with the thyroid, you must correct the hormone imbalance

- Proper adrenal tests are based on saliva, not blood

- Iodine loading will excrete the halogens (fluorine, chlorine, bromine) and other heavy metals

- It can cause severe detox symptoms, so you must go SLOW (can take anywhere from three months to many years)

- Iodine can help acne (though breakouts can initially worsen from bromine excretion)

- Sufficient iodine intake can result in resistance to parasitic infections

- Selenium, magnesium, and flax/fish oil should always accompany iodine loading

- Selenium is very important (can be obtained by eating one oz. of brazil nuts daily, garlic, astragalus)

- Magnesium is needed to help minimize detox reactions

- Iodine is carried from the intestines into the blood via essential fatty acids

- The most common symptom of thick/sluggish bile is bloating (caused by estrogen dominance)

- Eating beet roots and tops helps to thin bile.

- Sea salt is also important, as well as whole food complex B vitamins, vitamin A, and Vitamin C

- Sea salt does not contain enough iodine (for iodine supplementation)

Adrenal Fatigue

The symptoms of adrenal fatigue are very similar to those of hypothyroidism. Here is some extra information to help you better understand how the two are interrelated. The main symptoms of adrenal fatigue are:

Feeling tired despite sufficient hours of sleep
Insomnia
Weight gain
Depression
Hair loss
Acne
Reliance on stimulants like caffeine to keep you going
Cravings for carbohydrates or sugars as pick-me-ups
Cravings for salt
Poor immune function
Intolerance to cold

Sound familiar? They do if you have read the page on thyroid disease already. The chapter detailing my journey to wellness tells of my problems with both adrenal and thyroid dysfunction. You see, these two conditions are closely intertwined. The function of the adrenal glands is to give us energy for the "fight or flight" syndrome.

If you're running from the proverbial saber toothed tiger, you have no need at that moment for your food to be digested, or your liver to be filtering. All of your energy would be directed towards your heart, brain, arms and legs for fighting or fleeing.

The problem, of course, comes when we are constantly in this stress mode and the body never gets out of fight or flight. The adrenals are constantly pumping out adrenaline and cortisol until they are just depleted and can't produce any more.

Adrenals and thyroid connection

That's when the real problems begin. When your adrenals are working too hard, the thyroid can also suffer. It's a two-fisted hit, with one exacerbating the other.

High adrenaline output inhibits TSH (thyroid-stimulating hormone), which may or may not show up in a standard medical test. It also adversely impacts the conversion of T4 to T3 (which is the more active form of thyroid hormone), and decreases the function of T3 at the receptor level.

This is what happened to me. My body was not utilizing T3 properly, even though my TSH test showed normal.

The next step in the cascade is hypothyroidism, or an underactive thyroid. Hypothyroidism can lead to weight gain or difficulty losing weight, because it slows your metabolism.

It can also lead to a vicious cycle of being dead tired during the day to the point of needing a nap, or being almost unable to get out of bed in the morning. Sometimes, the person gets a "second wind" at around 6:00 PM, feeling wide awake. Of course, when they try to go to bed, they're suddenly "tired but wired" and cannot go to sleep. It's as if life has been turned upside down, or at least backwards.

This article from Dr. Mercola has more background information and outlines important steps to take, to help heal yourself. It can be found at this address: *http://articles.mercola.com/ sites/articles/archive/2002/11/20/reduce-stress.aspx*.

Your best bet is to find a good holistic, naturopathic doctor who can test you and find the right things to help you get well. Knowledge is the best way to regain your health and just being aware of what is causing the problem is a great step in the right direction.

Signs of Thyroid Disease

The following information is what alerted me to the signs of thyroid problems for myself when I happened to see it in a book I was reading. This list is taken from the book "The Coconut Diet" by Cherie Calbom.

These are symptoms of an underactive thyroid or hypothyroid condition. Give yourself 1 point for each symptom that applies to you.

1. Appetite problems - severely reduced or excessive

2. Bloating or indigestion after eating

3. Low body temperature (below 97.6 - resting)

4. Weight gain

5. Mucus accumulation

6. Hoarse throat

7. Cold hands and feet

8. Puffy eyes

9. Constipation

10. Decreased sweating

11. Dry mouth - drinking water doesn't help much

12. Intolerance to cold or heat

13. Poor digestion of animal products

14. Poor absorption of minerals

15. Sluggish lymph drainage

16. Swelling - ankles, eyelids, face, feet, hands, lymph nodes, throat

17. Spleen or liver problems

18. Calcium deficiency

19. Carpal tunnel syndrome

20. Left arm weakness

21. Muscle/joint problems - knees, elbows, etc.

22. Numbness in fingers

23. Stiff neck

24. Tenderness in lower ribs

25. Brittle nails

26. Grooves or ridges in nails

27. Thin, peeling nails

28. Slow-growing nails

29. White spots on nails (this can also be a zinc deficiency)

30. Fluttering in ears

31. Occasional stinging in eyes

32. Poor vision

33. Impotency
34. Loss of libido/low sex drive
35. Miscarriages
36. Premature deliveries
37. Spontaneous abortions
38. Stillbirths
39. Coarse, dry hair
40. Hair loss
41. Loss of hair on arms, underarms, legs, eyebrows, scalp
42. Elevated cholesterol
43. Enlargement of heart
44. Heart pain
45. Hypertension
46. Pain in diaphragm
47. Heart Palpitations
48. Impaired heart function
49. Slower heart rate
50. Sense of pressure (compression) on chest
51. PMS
52. Prolonged or heavy menstrual bleeding
53. Light menstrual flow
54. Shorter menstrual cycle
55. Bi-polarity (manic-depression)

Background Information

56. Depression

57. Difficulty concentrating

58. Emotionally unstable

59. Fatigue/lack of energy

60. Forgetfulness

61. Inability to "drag oneself from bed"

62. Lethargy

63. Nervousness

64. Restlessness

65. Shyness

66. Tendency to cry easily

67. Chronic mucus in head/nose (thyroid governs mucus production)

68. Shortness of breath

69. Difficulty drawing deep breath

70. Gasping of air occasionally

71. Intolerance to closed, stuffy rooms

72. Loss of smell

73. Need for fresh air

74. Sleep disturbances

75. Grinding teeth during sleep

76. Loss of hearing

A score of 20 points or more may be indicative of an under active thyroid.

Although this thyroid quiz may help you determine any signs of thyroid problems, ultimately the best method of diagnosis is clinical evaluation by a physician knowledgeable in thyroid health. See a physician who can treat your condition holistically.

Chapter 7

Resources

Directions to North Georgia Area Health Food Stores

Our local grocery stores, Kroger, Ingles and Food Lion, are trying hard to provide us with more organic and locally grown produce, and we should support them in this. Ingles has their organics spread out throughout the store within each section of foods, while Kroger concentrates theirs in the Nature's Market section.

Dawsonville's local health food store, Nature's Health, is located in the strip mall on the corner of Lumpkin Campground Road and Hwy. 53. While not offering food, it does carry Stevia and Xylitol, among other things.

Whole Foods and Natural Foods Warehouse

For those of us in the Dawsonville area, the closest marketplaces that carry a wide variety of organic and alternative foods are Whole Foods, and Natural Foods Warehouse. I'm aware that Whole Foods is often referred to as "whole paycheck," but you can either pay the grocer or pay the doctor, whichever you prefer. After all, what is your health worth?

I also know that it is quite a drive, but I go once a month and get everything I need to last the entire month. You need to think ahead so that you don't waste fuel as well as time. Good planning is essential. Go armed with a list of items to purchase and stick to that list.

Make a day of it and do all of your errands at once! If you are going to Atlanta down GA 400, Harry's Market (a Whole Foods store) is off of Exit 10 (Old Milton Parkway). Once you have exited, turn right (heading West) and go to Hwy 9/120, which is Main Street, then turn left. (This is the road right after Haynes Bridge Road.) Once you have turned, go straight until you pass Wills Road, and turn right at the next light—Upper Hembree Road.

Whole Foods (Harry's Market) is located about a quarter mile down this road on your left. You will see the signs. Be aware that once you enter Harry's parking lot, it is one way only.

Natural Foods Warehouse is on down GA 400 to Exit 8, which is Mansell Road. If heading South down 400, when you exit, you will turn left (East) and go one mile down Mansell to Old Alabama Road Connector.

Turn right onto Old Alabama and look for Spa Sydell on your left. Natural Foods Warehouse is a stand alone strip mall right behind it. Natural Foods Warehouse is just like the name implies, a warehouse. What they have varies from month to month, but there are many staple items that are offered consistently. If you find an item there, it is most likely the best price to be found anywhere. (Note: They do not accept checks.)

Going down 141 to Norcross

Both Natural Foods Warehouse and Whole Foods are also located on off of Hwy. 141 (Peachtree Parkway). If you are headed South down GA 400, take Exit 13. Turn left at the exit and drive for 10 miles (yes, it is exactly that far). You'll pass Parson's Road, and then the road after that is Wilson Road.

Immediately after Wilson Road, turn right into Medlock Bridge Shopping Center. (There is a sort of clock tower by the entrance.) Natural Foods Warehouse is directly in front of you. This location is their flagship store and it carries a wide variety of goods.

This is the purpose statement from their website which sums up their philosophy well:

We welcome you to the Natural Foods Warehouse family. Natural Foods Warehouse is an organic grocery store featuring dry grocery, freezer, perishable, vitamin/supplement, and health and beauty departments as well as 1,000's of the top selling items from the natural foods industry. At Natural Foods Warehouse, our goal is to bring you the top name brand items at the deepest possible discounts every day. We strive to give our customers a complete selection of name brand products as well as monthly featured specials. Natural Foods Warehouse requires no fee or membership to shop.

If you turn right out of the shopping center, go down to State Bridge Road (the next big intersection) and turn left, another Whole Foods store will be on your left, about a quarter mile down that road. From Natural Foods Warehouse to Whole Foods is a mile total, so it is easy to access both stores in one trip. By the way, it is only 1.6 miles further to this Whole Foods location from Dawsonville than it is to Harry's, so it's no big deal.

This Whole Foods store is more geared to convenience foods in that it has a lot of salad, soup and entree bars set up for people to buy food on the go. They have a seating area, too, so that you can eat it there like a fast food restaurant. They cater to a different group of people than the other store (Harry's) does.

Harry's will sometimes give you a 10% discount when you buy the whole package of organic meats as I suggest doing, because you are buying a lot of water within the package. The other Whole Foods will rarely do it, and then only if you insist on speaking to the manager. Even then, they do it grudgingly.

Of course, Atlanta has all sorts of great places for organic foods, such as Sevananda, Return to Eden, Life Grocery, and the Dekalb Farmer's market to name a few. Dawsonville's Farmer's Market is the epitome of local, and many times the produce is organically grown, even though not certified. Lelani's also carries organically grown but not certified produce.

In my opinion, it is well worth going to any of these places for fresh, minimally processed foods, which give you optimal health. See the Resources List on the following page for categories of individual items that you can purchase at either store.

Note: At press time for this book, I discovered that there are two more Natural Foods Warehouse Stores in the Atlanta area. I have not been to either one, and therefore cannot give you any directions, but here are the other two locations.

Store # 3
670 North Main Street
Alpharetta, GA 30009
770-619-0435

And Store # 4
12315 Crabapple Road
Alpharetta, GA 30004
770-772-0113

Resources List
For North Georgia Readers
As of January, 2011

N. F. = Natural Foods Warehouse
Harry's = Harry's Food Market or any Whole Foods store

I advocate going to Natural Foods Warehouse first, as they will normally have the lowest prices on items, and then going to Harry's or another Whole Foods store. Of course, I always try to support our local businesses as much as possible and only buy things in Atlanta that I can't get where I live.

Meats and fish

1. Whiteoak Pastures grass fed/finished beef – Publix; N. F.
2. Applegate Farms turkey, chicken and ham – Publix (in Gainesville at Thompson Bridge and Enota); Harry's
3. Applegate Farms turkey bacon – Ingles
4. Private Selection ground beef * – Kroger
5. Coleman uncured ham steak – Ingles or Harry's
6. Coleman chicken sausages – Ingles
7. Applegate Farms oven roasted chicken and turkey – Harry's
8. Wilshire Farms turkey ham – Harry's (has some sugar)
9. Salmon or tuna – order on-line from Vital choice

Dairy products

1. Redwood Hill Farm goat's milk yogurt – N. F. (pasteurized but not homogenized)
2. Cascade Fresh Activ8 yogurt ** – Harry's
3. Lifeway kefir ** – Ingles and Kroger
4. Raw Goat Milk mild cheddar cheese – N.F.
5. Organic Valley raw sharp and mild cheddar cheese – Kroger and Ingles

Nuts, dried fruit and seeds

1. Raw sunflower seeds – up front at Kroger's Natural Market beside the dairy section
2. Sulfite-free sundried tomatoes – Harry's (pasta aisle)
3. Sulfite-free dried fruit (cranberries) – Harry's
4. Organic nuts – baking goods section of Kroger

5. Organic raisins – dried fruit section of Kroger
6. Raw nuts and seeds – Harry's or N. F.
7. Medjool or Deglet dates – Harry's
8. Let's Do Organic shredded coconut and flakes –N. F.

Oils and grain substitutes

1. Extra virgin olive oil – best prices usually at N. F., Kroger, Harry's
2. Sesame oil – Ingles (with Thai food)
3. Organic sesame seed oil – Harry's or N. F.
4. Eden toasted sesame oil – Harry's or Food Lion
5. Fresh Shores coconut oil – Mercola.com (order online)
6. Fresh Shores coconut flour – Mercola.com (online)
7. Bob's Red Mill gluten-free or regular rolled oats – Harry's, N. F. or order online at Bob's Red Mill
8. Quinoa – Harry's
9. Arrowroot flour – Harry's
10. Almond flour – Kroger

Produce

1. Bagged Ready-to-use Kale – Ingles or Kroger
2. Bagged Earthbound Farms greens – Ingles
3. Clamshell packaged Private Selection organic greens – Kroger
4. Eat Smart bagged broccoli slaw and veggies – Kroger and Ingles
5. Fresh Express veggie packs – Kroger

Miscellaneous

1. Organic spices – Harry's, N. F., some at Kroger
2. Stevia – Harry's or N. F. for powdered versions or at Natural Health store
3. Xylitol – Harry's, or on-line through Emerald Forest
4. Luo Han Guo – order online
5. Sea Salt – Harry's or N. F.
6. Organic fair trade cocoa powder – Harry's or N. F.
7. Gluten-free pizza crust – Harry's (in frozen case)
8. Frozen organic cherries – Food Lion
9. Brown rice vinegar – Ingles, Harry's and N. F.
10. Flaxseeds – Kroger, Harry's or N. F.
11. Barlean's Forti-Flax – Harry's
12. Health from the Sun sprouted flax – N. F.
13. Raw tahini – Kroger, Harry's, N. F.

14. Organic Sesame tahini – Kroger
15. Miso Master organic miso – Harry's
16. Westbrae Natural organic mellow white miso – Kroger
17. Organic coconut milk in cans – Kroger, Harry's or N. F.
18. Regular coconut milk in cans – Ingles (Hispanic foods)
19. EnerG egg replacer – Harry's, N. F. or Kroger
20. Dr. Bronner's pure Castile soap – Kroger
21. Veggie Wash – Kroger (with eco cleaners in Natural Market area, and in produce)
22. Spiral Slicer – Joyce Chen (on internet)

* Private Selection is organic beef, but I don't know if it is grass-finished or not, a very important consideration.

** Both of these are pasteurized and homogenized (which you ideally want to avoid), but in a pinch, these are better than anything else at regular markets.

Please note that all of these items are subject to change. One store may discontinue an item while another store may pick it up. If you don't see an item, especially one that was formerly in stock, don't hesitate to ask a store employee or the manager if it is back-ordered, or if they have discontinued it. Many times the store will try to get it for you again if you do this.

ONLINE RESOURCES

Salmon or tuna – order on-line from Vital choice
Fresh Shores coconut oil – Mercola.com (order online)
Fresh Shores coconut flour – Mercola.com (online)
Bob's Red Mill gluten-free or regular rolled oats – order online at Bob's Red Mill
Xylitol – Harry's, or on-line through Emerald Forest
Luo Han Guo – order online
Spiral Slicer – Joyce Chen (on internet)

OTHER RESOURCES

Brenda Cobb, Living Foods Institute; www.LivingFoodsInstitute.com 800-844-9876
Brenda@livingfoodsinstitute.com; 404-607-1816 (Direct), 404-524-4488 (Main)

Jackie and Gideon Graff, Sprout Raw Food, www.rawfoodrevival.com;
email: rawfoodrevival@att.net

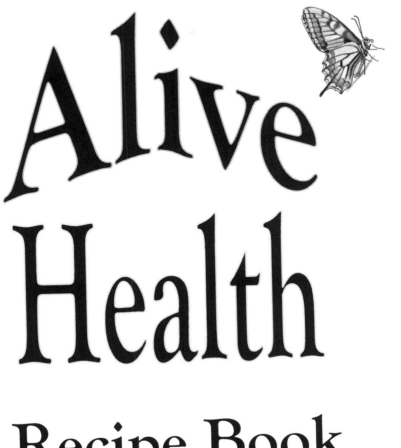

Recipe Book

PART TWO

RECIPES

Fun Fact: Per Barbara Pleasant in *The Southern Garden Advisor*, "Sweetpotato" has definitively been spelled as one word since before 2003. No exceptions!

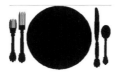

The Recipes

This section is the heart of the book. If you are already familiar with raw foods and Dr. Mercola's Nutritional Typing, you can just go ahead and dive in, and try some of the recipes. If not, I strongly urge you to read the first section of the book, to understand why the recipes use certain ingredients. At the very least, read through this section to get an idea.

All of the recipes here are wheat-free, gluten-free, sugar-free and artificial sweetener-free. Most are raw and many are vegan, for those who choose to go that route. I have given you an overview of different methods for gluten-free, so something somewhere should click for you. My goal is to give you quick and easy recipes that will allow you to have enough healthy food to eat for a week, while spending just a small portion of two days a week in the kitchen. It really and truly can be done, as I do it all the time.

But because we don't live in a vacuum, and holidays and special occasions come up, I have included a few more-time-consuming "party" recipes for those situations. Or if you just want to try something fancier, have a go at some of these. The Macadamia Mango Pie is somewhat hard to make, but it's so good that I had to include it. (It's one of my favorites.)

I have broken the sections down into Breakfast; Condiments, Gravies and Soups; Salad Dressings; Side Dishes; Main Meals; Crackers and Breads; Desserts, and finally, Beverages and Snacks. Many of the sections overlap and desserts can be snacks, breakfasts can be desserts, etc. They are mix and match in lots of categories.

What to Use

These recipes call for coconut oil, which is extremely good for you, and the natural sweeteners Stevia, Xylitol and Luo Han Guo, which we shorten to just Lo Han. One quarter teaspoon of Stevia or Lo Han is approximately equal to one quarter cup of sugar. Xylitol is used measure for measure the same as sugar. You have to use a lot of sweetener to counteract the bitterness of cocoa powder and regular plain yogurt. Remember, though, you can always add more, but you can't take it out if you put in too much.

I use only Dr. Mercola's whey protein because all of the others I've checked have been so vastly inferior. Please read the background chapters on all of these ingredients to better understand how and why I use them.

I recommend using a Vitamix blender and/or a food processor, but you can just use a good set of sharp knives and a lot of elbow grease, if necessary. A Saladacco makes great spaghetti "noodles" and it's a lot easier if you can get one. They are not very expensive.

Many of the items I use can only be bought at Natural Food Stores, or online, so in the first section of the book, I list places that have each item. I have gotten used to ordering lots of things online, which makes life a whole lot simpler.

Also, I make one trip a month down to Atlanta from my home up in the North Georgia mountains to buy things that I can't get locally. I always have a list and a plan of what food I am going to eat for a month, and I buy nothing but that.

Concerning meats, I buy grass-fed, grass-finished beef and pork from a local farm near me, by the cut, frozen, and take them home to my freezer. I take things out as I need them, such as four pork chops, thaw them overnight in the refrigerator, and cook up all four at one time. Then they are ready to grab and go as needed.

I buy packages of pre-cooked organic chicken and turkey from Whole Foods, bring them home and cut them up into three-ounce portions. Then I bag and freeze them in sets of two and take these out as needed. I buy free-range eggs and raw milk from other local sources, and get veggies from either my own garden, or local farmer's markets, as much as I can. Otherwise, they come from my local stores.

I make my own yogurt from raw milk and have strawberries and blueberries (and next year, raspberries) growing on my back deck. I buy raw cheeses from Whole Foods or Natural Foods Warehouse and even my local stores. Be aware that products in stores come and go, so if there is something you would like to have, ask the store manager to stock it. Chances are he or she will.

How to use the recipes

These recipes are designed for beginners up to advanced chefs, so there should again be something for nearly everyone. Some of the dishes are easy two-ingredient types and are therefore very simple. Others are more complicated and time consuming. All are good, or they wouldn't be in here.

The recipes are written with the ingredients listed in the order that they are to be used. However, my suggestion is to read the recipe through first to get a sense of it, and to be sure that you understand it. And please be sure to read the first section of this book for the reasoning behind why things are done the way they are. I assure you there is good, sound science behind all of it.

For the recipes that require cooking, be sure to pre-heat your oven first. I always wondered why they said to do that, as it seemed to me to be a waste of energy. Then I discovered why when I put an oven thermometer in to check on the temperature of my oven. (Ovens can be off by 25° or more, so it's a good idea to do this.)

Once the oven signals that it has reached the temperature you set it for, it takes a good 10 to 15 minutes longer before the entire oven heats up to the recorded temperature. If you put food in to be cooked before the whole oven is hot enough, you risk not getting it baked properly. That's the reason behind many culinary failures.

I recommend growing and using your own herbs, too, as this can greatly enhance the flavor of your dishes. They can be grown indoors or out, and are easy to cultivate.

Staple Items to Have On Hand

Here are the staples that I always keep in my pantry, most of which are organic. With these items around, and the addition of some fresh produce and a meat, I can quickly put together a meal to take with me or to eat right then.

1. Coconut oil
2. Coconut flour
3. Xylitol
4. Stevia
5. Lo Han
6. Raw macadamia nuts
7. Raw almonds
8. Cashews
9. Gluten-free oatmeal
10. Unsweetened coconut
11. Raisins
12. Chia seeds
13. Whey powder
14. Peanut butter

15. White and Apple Cider vinegar
16. Olive oil
17. Sun-dried tomatoes
18. Dried cranberries
19. Salba seeds
20. Cloves of garlic
21. Sesame oil
22. Toasted sesame oil
23. Balsamic vinegar
24. Sea salt
25. Brown rice vinegar
26. Aluminum-free baking powder
27. Baking soda
28. Various spices
29. Vanilla, lemon and almond extract
30. Cocoa powder
31. An assortment of tea bags
32. Raw cheeses

It's a good idea to always keep a good salad dressing on hand. That way if you are pressed for time, you can always grab some veggies from the produce section of your local store and put a home-made dressing on them for a quick meal. I've done that more times than I care to remember.

If you go to my website *www.HealthyEatingOnTheRun.com* and sign up for my newsletter, you can get a free Month of Menus which will give you exact details on how to have a month's worth of rotating meals to make and take with you. Try some of these Grab and Go Recipes now. Happy food fixing!

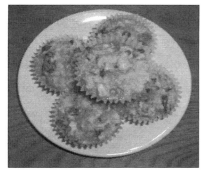
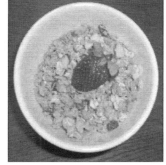
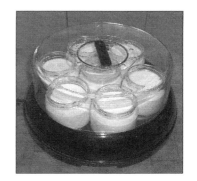
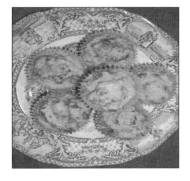

Breakfast

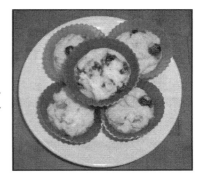
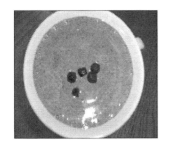
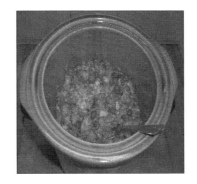
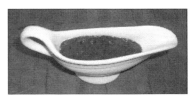
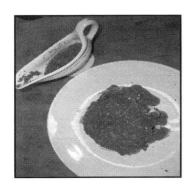
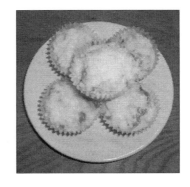
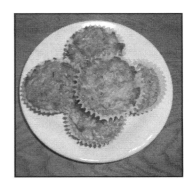

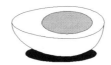

Healthy Eating Begins
With Breakfast

You've heard it before: Breakfast is the most important meal of the day. The statement bears repeating because it is absolutely true. Another statement that may be familiar is that one should "Eat breakfast like a king, lunch like a prince and dinner like a pauper." If you don't eat when you get up in the morning, you are more likely to overeat later in the day

This section gives you a lot of different choices—from a simple shake or cereal, to fruit rollups, pancakes, and muffins. There's a muffin recipe for each day of the week, and they are very portable.

A reminder: All of the recipes in this book are wheat-free, gluten-free, sugar-free and artificial sweetener-free. Many are dairy-free and vegan as well. If you would like to make your own nut milks, please see that section in Chapter 3 on page 52 for instructions.

All of them use coconut oil, and either coconut flour or oatmeal flour. There are three natural sweeteners that are used: Xylitol, Stevia and Luo Han Guo (or Lo Han), and there is a section in Chapter 3 on page 55 that gives you in-depth information on each of these sweeteners, if you are not familiar with them.

Helpful Tips for Making Granola Cereal

Oats are one of the few grains that are okay to eat as long as you are not gluten sensitive (see the section on Grains in Chapter 2, page 13). If you are, there is a brand that certifies their oats to be gluten-free—Bob's Red Mill. Otherwise, the regular, old-fashioned oats are the ones to use in the recipes, not the quick-cooking kind.

You can find these packages of gluten-free oats at Natural Foods Warehouse or Whole Foods in the Atlanta area. Otherwise, order them on-line from *www.bobsredmill.com.* They are fairly pricey, though.

Putting it all together

The first part of the recipe is just putting everything together in a big bowl. When you get to the second part of the recipe, however, you may need some extra help. There are pictures of the steps on my website at *www.HealthyEatingOnTheRun.com/granola-cereal.html.*

First, melt the coconut oil by putting the jar into a pan of simmering water on the stove. Coconut oil is solid at temperatures under 72°F. From 72° to 76°, it is somewhat creamy in texture, and its melting point is above 76°.

Then melt the peanut butter by repeating the process, using a two-cup capacity Pyrex (glass) measuring cup, with one cup of organic Valencia peanut butter in it. This acts like a double boiler to keep the peanut butter from scorching. Trust me on this, burned peanut butter is not very appetizing, so be patient.

While you are waiting for the peanut butter to melt (it does help to have it at room temperature before you start), pour the melted coconut oil into it. This helps the peanut butter melt faster. Still, the process will take anywhere from 30 minutes to more than an hour.

Add the Stevia and vanilla to the melted mixture and stir until well blended. Then pour it over the dry ingredients, mix it together well, and you're done!

How to prepare your cereal for eating

The day before you want to have some of the cereal, pour some plain, preferably home-made, yogurt over it (about three heaping tablespoons, or a small jar of it), and cover it with plastic wrap. Place it in the refrigerator overnight (for 12-24 hours) to get the phytates neutralized before eating it the next day. (See "Soaking Grains" in Chapter 2, page 15, for why.)

It will be somewhat runny after the yogurt is added. When you take it out to eat it the next day, however, it will be very thick. You can add some raw milk, coconut milk, Almond milk, or Rice milk to bring it to the consistency you prefer.

Put in some Stevia or Lo Han sweetener to taste and enjoy a healthy eating treat! (Be sure to wait and put the sweetener in right before you eat it.) You can also add some fruit of your choice as well, such as strawberries, blueberries, etc. Whatever you do, please do not use sugar! The section on Sugar in Chapter 2, page 17, will explain why I say this.

I eat a bowl of this cereal as a "dessert" just about every day. So, as soon as I finish a bowl, I wash it out, put more cereal in, and add the yogurt to it for the next day. If I'm not going to be around the next day, for whatever reason, I don't set it up. Instead, I wait until I know I will be in and able to eat it. It is a wonderful dessert!

Best bet for breakfast

My breakfast of choice, especially in warmer months, is a smoothie. It is really easy to make. If you are pressed for time in the mornings, you can get the ingredients ready the night before and just throw them in the blender when you get up the next day.

You can purchase a neat traveling mug and take your smoothie with you if you really need to. I have taken mine when doing a fasting blood test at a lab, and it works really well. The mugs are available at my local Kroger and are around $10.00 each, sometimes being on sale for around $6.96 if you want to keep checking back. (See a picture of the mug I use on my website at *www.HealthyEatingOnTheRun.com/healthy-breakfast.html.*)

A thermal mug also works great for taking your smoothie with you. Some of them even have holes for a straw, as does my mug. But beware...drinking anything through a straw will put lines on your lips, just like smoking cigarettes does! I always use a spoon at home, so I can savor every mouthful.

How to make a smoothie

The ingredients are basically the same, and I rotate the frozen fruit between blueberries, strawberries, and cherries, with peaches or mangoes occasionally, just for variety. Any kind of frozen *organic only* fruit will do.

For the protein, I use only Dr. Mercola's Pro-Optimal Whey™, his Whey Protein with Aminogen™, or his newest product, Miracle Whey™. Please do not use anything other than this brand as all of the others are vastly inferior. (There is a comparison of these and three other brands in Chapter 3 on page 38.) Dr. Mercola's six flavors taste wonderful, too!

For those of you who prefer not to use milk derivatives, Pea Protein is a good substitute. Do NOT use any soy products. Unless it is fermented, soy is not a health food and will do major harm to your body.

Pea Protein is available at most local health food stores including Nature's Health in Dawsonville, where I live. It can also be ordered from Dr. Mercola's site. He frequently gives free shipping specials. I personally don't care for the taste of pea protein, though.

For the yogurt, I typically make my own from raw goat's milk. Raw milk is far better for you than pasteurized for many reasons, and goat's milk is superior to cow's milk since it is closer to human milk. For my local readers, I will be glad to give you a source for raw goat's milk or cow's milk if you will contact me. Eating some type of probiotics daily is an excellent health enhancer.

A tablespoon of ground Salba or chia seeds is a wonderful addition to smoothies, especially if you are vegan or vegetarian. They are gluten-free, have relatively few calories, and are reasonably priced.

You can also add in a tablespoon of flaxseeds, although I think that is a little bit redundant if you are using Salba or chia seeds. A tablespoon of raw almond butter is a yummy addition but be aware that both of these significantly raise the calorie level of the shake.

If you are not having any problems with your weight, flaxseeds and almond butter are great additions to your smoothie that will keep you satisfied for a long time afterwards.

I've been known to easily go five or six hours before being hungry for lunch, which was unheard of, for me, before I changed my way of eating. I used to have hypoglycemia and was not fun to be around when I didn't have anything to eat at the time I needed it. Even I didn't like being around me!

Making yogurt

Yogurt is very easy to make. I use Yolife brand yogurt maker from Tribest as it has a larger cover for making bigger batches, if you so desire. It comes with seven ½ cup containers. I use one container in my smoothie, if I'm not using regular raw milk. If I am using store-bought yogurt, I put in three heaping tablespoons of it.

Since it is plain yogurt, you will need to add some kind of sweetener. Please do not ever use any of the artificial sweeteners (such as Splenda, Equal, or NutraSweet) as they do devastating things to your health. Ditto for high fructose corn syrup.

Stevia, Xylitol or Luo Han Guo are the best natural sweetener alternatives to use. My preference is either Stevia or Luo Han Guo. I feel that Xylitol is best used in baking to give bulk to baked goods, the same way sugar does.

Using raw eggs

After I have put all of the ingredients in the blender and mixed them together, the last thing that I add is a raw egg. Yes, I know, you are probably saying "Major yuck!" right now, but raw eggs are great nutrition for you.

If you put the egg in slowly to preserve the integrity of the yolk, you will never know it is in there. Simply turn the blender on to the lowest setting just long enough to take the egg down into the mix and then immediately shut the motor off.

Please read the information on how to test eggs in Chapter 4 (under Raw Eggs on page 69) before adding one to your smoothie. There are obviously some precautions that you need to take to make sure the egg is safe to eat, but the rewards are definitely worth it.

If you haven't noticed already, everything that goes into this smoothie is raw food. There are very good reasons for that; it's easier to do that way, and healthier for you, too.

Using a Vitamix

I'd like to offer a recommendations on the proper blender to use. You can use a regular one, but I highly recommend that you splurge on a Vitamix. You will never regret it, and will use it constantly if you decide to follow this way of healthy eating.

A Vitamix is a powerful tool that can help you make the most of organic foods by preserving all of the nutrients. Recipes are easy to make, and the machine is fun to use, as well.

If you use a regular blender, be aware that frozen cherries, even though they are supposed to be pitted, frequently will have pieces that were missed, or sometimes even whole pits. A normal blender cannot handle this and will break. So, you may want to forgo using cherries.

After you break enough regular blenders, you'll probably decide that a Vitamix is a good investment. These are powerhouses, like a blender on steroids, that can take almost any kind of abuse. I advocate the one with variable speeds because there are many cases where you will need a low speed (adding raw eggs, making mayonnaise, etc.).

And now, it's time to go play in the kitchen!

Morning Wake-up Shake

In a Vitamix blender, add all of the following ingredients:

> ½ to one frozen banana, depending on size
> ½ cup frozen fruit (blueberry, strawberry, peach, etc.)
> ½ to ⅔ cup raw milk, Rice milk, Almond milk or yogurt (plain)
>   *(Put in a little milk to prevent motor strain if using yogurt)*
> 1 tablespoon ground Salba, chia or flaxseeds
>   *(If bought whole, grind in a dedicated coffee grinder)*
> 1 tablespoon raw almond butter, if desired
> 1 scoop of Dr. Mercola's Protein powder (choice of flavors)
> Stevia, Luo Han Guo or Xylitol to taste if using yogurt

1. Mix together in Vitamix (use tamper if necessary)
2. Add in a raw egg *slowly* after all of the other ingredients have been blended. First test the egg (see page 71) for safety.
3. Pour into a mug or bowl and enjoy! Use a travel mug and take, if needed.

I like to use chocolate protein powder with blueberries, strawberry with strawberries, and vanilla with any of the other fruits, but you may choose any combination you like. See the text on "How to Make a Smoothie," page 110, for details on the ingredients.

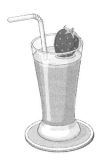

Sweet Breakfast Granola

(Makes about 22 servings, ⅔ cup each)

8 cups rolled oats
1 cup unsweetened flaked coconut
1 cup your choice of nuts (except walnuts)
1 cup of raisins
4 tablespoons Salba, chia or sesame seeds
4 teaspoons cinnamon

1. Mix all ingredients together in a large bowl
2. Heat the following ingredients gently in a 2-cup Pyrex measuring cup that is sitting in a pot of simmering water, over medium heat:

   1 cup peanut butter (Valencia is a sweeter kind of peanut)
   ½ cup coconut oil
   1 teaspoon Stevia powder, to taste
   2 teaspoons vanilla extract or vanilla powder

3. Pour the mixture over the dry ingredients and blend until well mixed.
4. Store in an airtight container in the fridge and eat with raw milk or yogurt.
5. You can also add your choice of fresh fruit (strawberries, blueberries, banana, etc.) to your serving.

Each serving of cereal should be soaked for 12-24 hours in an acidulated medium (like yogurt) in order to neutralize the anti-nutrients before consuming.

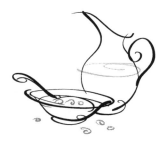

Slow Cooker Porridge

Makes ten ½ cup servings

1 cup whole-grain brown rice
Pinch of Stevia or Lo Han
1 tablespoon unsalted butter
½ teaspoon sea salt
½ teaspoon cinnamon
1 cup finely chopped apple, unpeeled
½ cup raisins
½ cup chopped walnuts or almonds
4 cups of water

1. Grease a 3.5 to 4 quart slow cooker with coconut oil or butter.
2. Place all ingredients in the crock pot and mix well.
3. Cover and cook on low 8 hours, or overnight.
4. Stir before serving.

This is great to have in the winter time for a hot breakfast if you don't want to go raw. Set it up the night before and you'll have a divinely smelling breakfast ready for you when you get up. It's perfect for when you have guests over. You may substitute old-fashioned rolled oatmeal for the brown rice.

Breakfast

Protein Pancakes

Makes 8 pancakes

2 scoops Dr. Mercola's Whey Protein. your choice of flavors
⅓ cup coconut flour
¼ teaspoon salt
1 teaspoon aluminum-free baking powder
2 large eggs (or 3 small), gently beaten
¾ cup raw milk
2 tablespoons cold water
🕐 **2 tablespoons melted coconut oil, plus some to grease the pan**

1. Sift whey, coconut flour, baking powder, and salt together.
2. Mix all remaining ingredients in another bowl and slowly add to dry ingredients, whisking until smooth.
3. Let stand at room temperature for 15 minutes.
4. Oil the bottom of a heavy skillet or griddle with coconut oil; set over medium heat. It's ready when a drop of water dances on the surface.
5. Stir batter and pour ¼ cup into 4" circles, allowing space between them.
6. Cook until bubbles form on the surface and the edges are dry. Turn and cook the other side.
7. Serve immediately with strawberry or blueberry syrup (next recipe) or with maple syrup or honey.
8. The pancakes can also be frozen for you to have at a later date.

🕐 *Indicates something that needs to be done ahead of time*

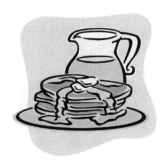

Strawberry Syrup

1 cup strawberries, washed and stems removed
1 teaspoon lemon juice
Lo Han or Stevia to taste

1. Place all ingredients in blender and blend until smooth.

Luo Han Guo (shortened to Lo Han) is best to use in syrup because it is derived from fruit and has a fruity flavor that adds to it. A little goes a long way, so start with just the tip of a regular teaspoon. You can always add more.

Blueberry Syrup

1 cup blueberries
1 teaspoon lemon juice
Lo Han or Stevia to taste

1. Place all ingredients in blender and blend until smooth.

This syrup may thicken if not eaten immediately. The pectin in the blueberries causes the jelling, If it occurs, just blend again, or thin with a little water.

The syrups can be used over ice cream or pancakes.

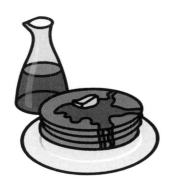

Breakfast

Homemade Yogurt
Makes 7-8 servings

1 quart (4 cups) fresh, raw cow or goat's milk *(at room temperature)*
3 tablespoons of yogurt "culture" *(at room temperature)*

1. Put the milk into a container big enough to stir it easily.
2. Add the 3 Tbsp. of yogurt (using a plastic measure) from either a previously made batch (up to five "generations" of use) or from store-bought yogurt with live active cultures. Make sure the container doesn't just say "made with" cultures but rather "contains" live, active cultures. *(You can use packaged cultures but I haven't had good luck with any of those.)*
3. Use a non-metal whisk to blend the culture thoroughly into the milk. For some reason, metal utensils cause the yogurt to not set well.

Using a yogurt making machine, such as Yolife, is the easiest way. In this case, you would use the seven jars included with it. If using the machine, fill up each jar with the cultured milk *and leave the lids off.*

Put them in the machine and plug it in, noting on the cover when eight hours will be up. The machine will heat it to 90°F and in 8-12 hours, you will have yummy, creamy yogurt as raw as you can get it to be. See the section "How to Make Yogurt" for alternative how-to information.

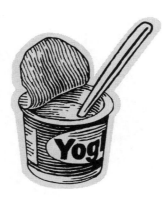

Alive Health Recipe Book

Fruit Leather Crepes
(Servings depend on quantity of fruit used)

Made with very ripe fruit—bananas, strawberries, blueberries, etc.

1. Take any fruit that is overripe and puree it in a blender.
2. Spread out onto a Teflex sheet and place in a dehydrator.
3. Dehydrate at 105°F for 6 to 8 hours.
4. Peel the leathers off the Teflex sheet halfway through, and leave them on the mesh sheet for the remainder of the time.
5. When done, take the leather off the mesh and cut it into sections about 4"x6" or so.
6. Add a filling of your choice, and roll up. Serve.

For fillings, you can use fruit, sour cream, cream cheese, etc., and top it with either blueberry or strawberry syrup if desired. Let your imagination and the leftovers in your fridge be your guide.

If you don't have a dehydrator, you can put the crepes in your oven on the lowest setting. Leave the door open a bit. They won't be raw, but they will firm up. Watch to see how long you should leave them in. Ovens vary greatly.

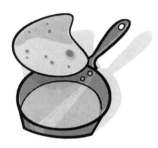

Banana Nut Muffins

Makes 6 muffins

3 eggs
2 tablespoons butter or coconut oil, melted
½ ripe banana, mashed
3 tablespoons Xylitol
¼ teaspoon salt
½ teaspoon vanilla
¼ cup sifted coconut flour
¼ teaspoon baking powder
¼ cup walnuts or pecans, chopped

1. Preheat oven to 400°F.
2. Blend together eggs, butter, banana, Xylitol, salt, and vanilla.
3. Combine coconut flour and baking powder; sift into the other ingredients
4. Mix thoroughly until there are no lumps.
5. Fold in nuts.
6. Pour into greased or lined muffin tins.
7. Bake at 400° for 18 minutes, or until browned on top.

🕐 *Indicates something that needs to be done ahead of time*

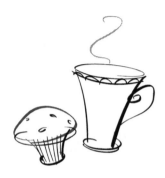

Blueberry Cranberry Muffins

Makes 6 muffins—they're great for the 4th of July!

3 eggs
🕐 **2 tablespoons butter, melted**
2 tablespoons coconut or whole milk
3 tablespoons Xylitol
¼ teaspoon salt
¼ teaspoon vanilla
¼ teaspoon baking powder
¼ cup sifted coconut flour
¼ cup dry blueberries
¼ cup frozen cranberries *(may be found with frozen vegetables)*

1. Preheat oven to 400°F.
2. Blend together eggs, butter, milk, Xylitol, salt, and vanilla.
3. Combine coconut flour with baking powder and sift into batter.
4. Thoroughly mix batter until there are no more lumps.
5. Fold in blueberries and cranberries. *(Make sure blueberries are dry. If they have been rinsed, dry them before adding to the batter.)*
6. Pour batter into greased or lined muffin cups.
7. Bake at 400°F for 16-18 minutes.

🕐 *Indicates something that needs to be done ahead of time*

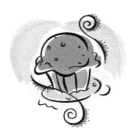

Breakfast

Salmon Sausage Muffins
Makes 6 muffins

1 Vital Choice Italian Salmon Sausage patty (or other sausage)
3 eggs
2 tablespoons coconut oil or butter, melted
½ teaspoon salt
¼ teaspoon onion powder
3 tablespoons sifted coconut flour
¼ teaspoon baking powder
¼ cup sharp cheddar cheese, grated

1. Preheat oven to 400°F.
2. Lightly cook the sausage in coconut oil in a frying pan, just enough to get it to come apart easily and thaw it out.
3. Cut sausage up into small pieces and set aside.
4. Blend together eggs, oil, salt, and onion powder.
5. Combine coconut flour and baking powder, and sift into batter.
6. Stir batter until there are no lumps.
7. Fold in sausage and most of the cheese, reserving a bit for the tops.
8. Spoon batter into lined or greased muffin cups.
9. Sprinkle the rest of the cheese on top of muffins.
10. Bake at 400° for 15 minutes, or until browned and cheese is melted.

Indicates something that needs to be done ahead of time

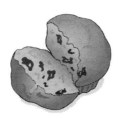

Zucchini Muffins

Makes 6 muffins

3 eggs
🕐 1 tablespoon butter or coconut oil, melted
3 tablespoons Xylitol
¼ teaspoon vanilla
¼ teaspoon salt
½ teaspoon cinnamon
⅛ teaspoon ground mace
⅓ cup sifted coconut flour
¼ teaspoon baking powder
½ cup shredded zucchini
¼ cup nuts

1. Preheat oven to 400°F.
2. Combine eggs, butter or oil, vanilla, salt, cinnamon, and mace.
3. Mix Xylitol in slowly to ensure even distribution.
4. Sift coconut flour and baking soda together and add to egg mixture.
5. Stir until there are no lumps left.
6. Fold in the shredded zucchini.
7. Fold in nuts.
8. Pour into muffin cups and bake at 400° for 18-20 minutes.

🕐 *Indicates something that has to be done ahead of time*

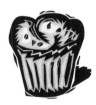

Breakfast

Carrot Walnut Muffins
Makes 6 muffins

🕐
3 eggs
2 tablespoons butter, melted
3 tablespoons Xylitol
¼ teaspoon salt
¼ teaspoon vanilla
¼ cup sifted coconut flour
¼ teaspoon baking powder
½ cup shredded carrot
¼ cup walnuts (or pecans), chopped
¼ cup raisins

1. Preheat oven to 400°F.
2. Blend together eggs, butter, Xylitol, salt, and vanilla.
3. Combine coconut flour with baking powder and whisk into batter until there are no lumps.
4. Fold in carrots, nuts and raisins.
5. Fill greased muffin cups with batter.
6. Bake at 400° for 16 minutes, or until browned on top.

🕐 *Indicates something that must be done ahead of time*

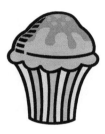

Apple Nut Muffins
Makes 6 muffins

3 eggs
🕐 **3 tablespoons butter, melted**
3 tablespoons Xylitol
¼ teaspoon salt
¼ teaspoon vanilla
¼ teaspoon almond extract
¼ cup sifted coconut flour
¼ teaspoon baking powder
½ cup finely chopped apple
¼ cup chopped walnuts or pecans
¼ teaspoon cinnamon

1. Preheat oven to 400°F.
2. In a bowl, combine eggs, butter, Xylitol, salt, vanilla, and almond extract.
3. Sift coconut flour and baking powder and add to wet ingredients.
4. Stir until there are no lumps.
5. Fold in apple, cinnamon, and nuts.
6. Pour batter into greased muffin cups.
7. Bake at 400° for 16-18 minutes, or until browned on top.

🕐 *Indicates something that needs to be done ahead of time*

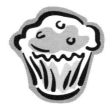

Breakfast

Blueberry Muffins

Makes 6 muffins

3 eggs
3 tablespoons butter, melted
3 tablespoons Xylitol
¼ teaspoon salt
¼ teaspoon vanilla
¼ teaspoon almond extract
¼ cup sifted coconut flour
¼ teaspoon baking powder
½ cup fresh blueberries (don't use frozen)

1. Preheat oven to 400°F.
2. In a bowl, combine eggs, butter, Xylitol, salt, vanilla, and almond extract.
3. Sift coconut flour and baking powder and add to wet ingredients.
4. Stir until there are no lumps.
5. Make sure blueberries are dry, then fold them into the batter.
6. Pour batter into greased muffin cups.
7. Bake at 400° for 16-18 minutes or until browned on top.
8. Cool on a rack and serve.

Indicates something that needs to be done ahead of time

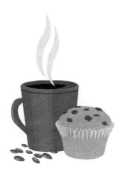

Alive Health Recipe Book

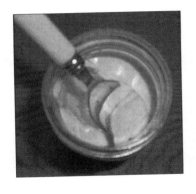
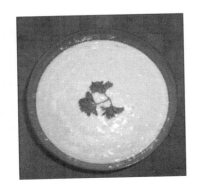
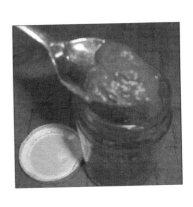

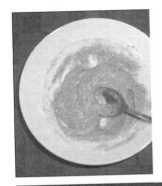

Condiments, Gravies and Soups

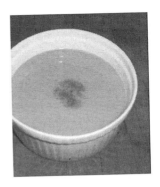

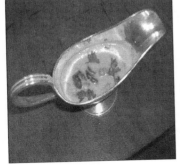
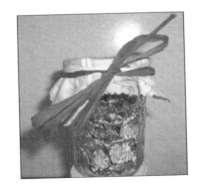
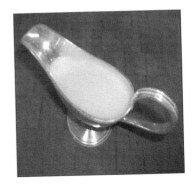

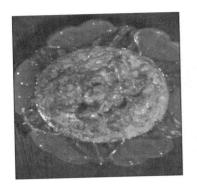
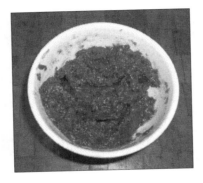
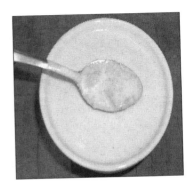

Condiments, Gravies and Soups

The recipes in this section offer substitutions for condiments that people use all the time. Most store-bought ketchup and mustard, for example, are full of nutritionally-undesirable fillers and add-ins that I would not want my family to eat. To see what I mean, take a look at some of the labels on products that may be in your refrigerator right now. (The same goes for gravy mixes.)

The soups can be eaten either raw and cold, or warmed up gently. I eat mostly raw, even in the winter, but there are times I just need something warm. So don't feel you are cheating if you heat them. Pumpkin is introduced in this section, so here's some information on it:

How to Make Raw Pumpkin

Raw pumpkin can be used in the recipes instead of canned, and is much better for you. (Be sure to buy "pie" or "cooking" pumpkins, not the type used for jack-o-lanterns.) Once you get your pumpkin home, cut it into quarters and scoop out the seeds. Remove the skin using either a knife or a potato peeler. This is admittedly the most difficult, time-consuming part, but once it's done, you have lots of pumpkin that you can use in many recipes.

Cut the pumpkin into small pieces and put it in a food processor to chop it very fine, or puree it in a Vitamix blender. Then you're ready to use it in your recipe. Now what are you going to do with all of the excess? Well, pureed pumpkin can be frozen. Chopped can be dehydrated for future use. Either way, you won't have to bother with preparing another pumpkin again (until next year, that is).

To dehydrate, chop the pumpkin into 1" cubes and place on a dehydrator shelf using the Teflex sheet. Dehydrate for 6-8 hours (overnight) at 105°F in an Excalibur dehydrator. Then put it into recycled jars of any type, not necessarily canning jars.

Label them with the date. When ready to use again, reconstitute by soaking them in hot water for 45 minutes. Almost a whole pumpkin will fit into a very small jar. ¼ cup dried pumpkin equals 2 cups reconstituted. (See what I mean?)

How to Use Raw Pumpkin

Be sure to check out the recipe for raw pumpkin pie. It is super easy to make, after you have prepared the pumpkin as previously instructed. People raved about the pie when I served it, and I didn't tell them until afterward that it was raw. The Pumpkin Oatmeal and Banana Bread are both pretty awesome, too, and give you a comfort-food feeling while you're eating them.

How to Dry Pumpkin Seeds

Clean the seeds that you remove from the pumpkin really well to get all the strings off. Then dry them spread out on paper towels for two weeks, changing the paper towels as needed. They are dry when you can crack them by bending them with your thumb. Store in a cool, dry place in an air-tight container.

Mine got mold on them when I dried them in the dehydrator, so this is a better method. Thanks to Jean Schilling of Country Home Kennels for the info!

How to Cook Pumpkin

If you would rather cook your field or store-bought pumpkin, here's how to do it. Preheat the oven to 350°F. Rest the pumpkin on its side and cut off the top, including the stem. Cut the pumpkin in half, from top to bottom, then into quarters and finally into eighths.

Remove the seeds and pulp. (You can wash, dry and roast the seeds in the oven and then sprinkle with a little salt for a healthy snack.) Bake the pumpkin for 45 minutes, or until fork-tender. Remove and let cool. Scrape the pumpkin meat from the shell (the skin will likely peel right off) and puree in a blender. Strain to remove the stringy pieces. Then use or freeze for later use.

Mayonnaise
Makes approximately 1½ cups (about 12 servings)

1 whole egg (test eggs first—see page 70-71)
2 egg yolks
2 teaspoons prepared ground mustard (in the spice aisle)
1 tablespoon lemon juice
½ teaspoon sea salt
¼ teaspoon white pepper
½ cup coconut oil, melted
½ cup grapeseed oil

1. Put the eggs, mustard, lemon juice, salt, and pepper into the Vitamix.
2. Turn it on low, and start adding the oils *very slowly*. It should take about two minutes to add all the oil.
3. This should last over a month in the refrigerator, and be fairly easy to spread, although you may need to let it warm up just a little. I suggest writing the date on it when you first make it.

🕐 *Indicates something that needs to be done ahead of time*

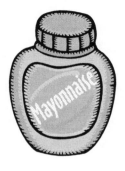

Barbecue Sauce
Makes 2 cups

🕐 **2 cups sun-dried tomatoes, soaked 1-2 hours (reserve soak water)**

🕐 **8 pitted dates, soaked 1 hour**

🕐 **½ cup red onion, chopped (put in the freezer for 10 minutes before cutting)**

1 tablespoon Extra Virgin Olive Oil

1 tablespoon lemon juice

½ tablespoon dried rosemary or 1 tablespoon fresh

½ tablespoon dried thyme or 1 tablespoon fresh

1 teaspoon paprika

½ teaspoon cayenne pepper

1. Put all of the ingredients into a Vitamix blender or food processor.
2. Puree them together until there are no chunks left.
3. Add some of the soak water as needed to get the right consistency.
4. Use on your favorite meat for grilling.

This keeps for a week in the refrigerator, so only make enough to use at one time. (It tastes wonderful. I know you'll want to use it often.)

🕐 *Indicates something that needs to be done ahead of time*

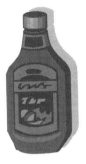

Condiments, Gravies and Soups

Individual Servings of Ketchup

Store-bought ketchup is full of all kinds of undesirable ingredients. Here is a recipe to make it yourself so that you have control over what goes into it.

1 tablespoon organic tomato puree (or paste if unavailable)
¾ teaspoon apple cider vinegar
Dash of Stevia (to taste)
¼ teaspoon garlic, finely minced
Pinch of cayenne (optional)
¼ teaspoon fresh basil, chopped fine
¼ teaspoon onion powder (optional) (*I don't use it if making ketchup for the Salmon salad because I already have onion in there.*)

Whisk all together in a small bowl. Makes one serving.
Use this for the Salmon salad recipe or wherever else you desire.

To make it easier if you need a larger amount, here is the **recipe doubled**.

2 tablespoons organic tomato puree (or paste)
1½ teaspoons apple cider vinegar
⅛ teaspoon Stevia (to taste)
½ teaspoon garlic, finely minced
Pinch of cayenne (optional)
½ teaspoon fresh basil, chopped fine
½ teaspoon onion powder (optional)

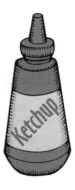

Mustard
Makes approximately 12 teaspoons

¼ **cup ground mustard (in the spice aisle)**
🕐 **3 tablespoons boiling water**
1 tablespoon apple cider vinegar
¼ **teaspoon sea salt**
Dash of Stevia, to taste

1. Combine all ingredients in a small bowl.
2. Stir until smooth; should be the consistency of a paste.
3. Store in the refrigerator, in a small glass jar with a lid.

This recipe can be substituted for prepared mustard in any of the recipes in this book. It eliminates the junk that is found in most brands of prepared mustards.

A word of caution: This makes a Dijon style, pretty spicy mustard. To tame it down, add more Stevia and/or let it sit for a couple of days.

🕐 *Indicates something that needs to be done ahead of time*

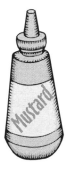

White Gravy
Makes 1 cup

1 cup raw milk of your choice (cow, goat, almond, rice, etc.)
1 tablespoon arrowroot
2 tablespoons butter
¼ teaspoon salt
⅛ teaspoon pepper

1. Mix arrowroot into cold milk in a saucepan.
2. Place over medium heat, stirring constantly.
3. Add butter, salt, and pepper.
4. Continue stirring and heating it gently until you reach desired thickness.
5. Remove from heat at that point and it is ready to serve.

You can buy arrowroot powder from Bob's Red Mill online, or get it at some organic markets. It comes from the root of a tropical plant and is tasteless. It needs to be mixed into cold liquid, and as it heats up, it starts to thicken. It is a great substitute for flour or cornstarch, the latter of which is nearly always a product of genetically modified corn.

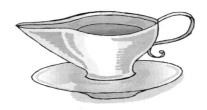

Mushroom Gravy
Makes approximately 2 cups

8-ounces fresh mushrooms, sliced
1 cup onion, finely chopped
1 tablespoon arrowroot flour
1½ cups raw milk of your choice (coconut milk is sweeter)
2 tablespoons butter
2 teaspoons salt
¼ teaspoon pepper
1 teaspoon fresh parsley
2 tablespoons coconut oil

1. Sauté mushrooms and onions in 2 tablespoons of coconut oil until tender.
2. Combine arrowroot flour with milk and stir into mixture.
3. Add butter, salt, and pepper.
4. Simmer, stirring frequently, for about 15 minutes.
5. Add parsley at the end of cooking.
6. Serve over roast beef, or meatballs, or even zucchini "noodles."

This is a great sauce for Swedish meatballs.

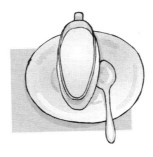

Pumpkin Coconut Soup

Makes 8 servings

2 lbs. pumpkin or butternut squash (4 cups), peeled and diced
1 cup onions
3 cloves of garlic
4 cups vegetable stock
1 can (14 oz.) coconut milk or 1¾ cups
1 teaspoon nutmeg or pumpkin pie spice
Dash of Stevia or Lo Han
Salt and pepper to taste

1. Place pumpkin in a pot with a few inches of water and cook until tender.
2. Sautee the onion and garlic in either butter or coconut oil
3. Put pumpkin in Vitamix blender along with the sautéed onions and garlic.
4. Add vegetable stock, milk, nutmeg, and sweetener, and puree until smooth.
5. Add salt and pepper to taste. Serve.

You can substitute two cans of pumpkin for the raw. If you plan to eat the soup cold, skip Step 1 and use the pumpkin raw. If it's cold outside and you need something warm, then cook the pumpkin according to the recipe, and gently reheat leftovers as needed.

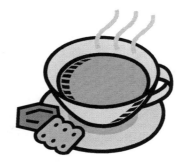

Dehydrated Soup

You can make your own soup fixings and store in any clean, recycled jar. These make great gifts. Here's an example of what to include.

Carrots
Onions
Green beans
Celery
Dried beans (air-dried in the pod, not in the dehydrator)

Dehydrate the vegetables (except the beans) then put everything into the jar. Cut out a piece of scrap cloth, if desired, and put over the lid with a rubber band. Tie a piece of ribbon or raffia around that to dress it up, especially if it is going to be a gift.

To me, there's nothing better than a gift from your garden, especially for your non-gardening friends. Include the instructions for use on the side of the jar.

When ready to make the soup, use about 1/4 cup of ingredients to 2 cups of water and simmer on the stove to your level of doneness. (I like mine still crunchy.) If you like meat, add small pieces, plus seasonings to taste.

This is a great soup for those cold winter days when you need something warm to eat. You don't have to be raw all year long, but try to eat raw as much as possible.

138

Tomato Basil Celery Soup
Makes four 16 oz. servings

🕐 **1 cup pine nuts, soaked 8 hours or overnight**
1¾ cups water
2-3 cloves garlic (can leave skins on)
¼ teaspoon crushed red pepper
🕐 **1 cup sun-dried tomatoes (soaked 1-2 hours to soften)**
6 cups tomatoes
🕐 **1 small Vidalia onion (put in freezer for 10 minutes before cutting)**
1 cup fresh basil
2 teaspoons sea salt
2-3 celery stalks

1. Place the nuts, water, red pepper flakes, and garlic in a Vitamix and blend.
2. Add soaked dried tomatoes and blend until smooth (*hold on to Vitamix while doing this as it tends to jump around*).
3. Pour into a large serving bowl.
4. Place basil in food processor and chop.
5. Add onion to processor and chop.
6. Add tomatoes to processor and blend it all together.
7. Stir mixture from food processor into creamy ingredients in serving bowl.
8. Chop the celery into small bits and stir into bowl along with the salt.
9. Serve cold or warmed slightly (in a dehydrator or double boiler on stove).

🕐 *Indicates something that needs to be done ahead of time*

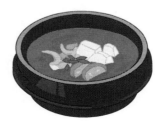

Alive Health Recipe Book

Broccoli Cheese Soup
Makes 2 cups

1 cup raw milk of your choice, warmed but not hot
⅓ cup raw organic cheddar cheese
1 cup broccoli, barely steamed (*counteracts goitrogenic properties*)
¼ cup onion
1 teaspoon arrowroot (*for thickening*)

1. Heat milk gently on the stove, enough to warm it but not kill the enzymes.
2. Steam broccoli in a steamer (*metal piece designed to go into a pan with a few inches of water underneath it*). If you don't have one, put the broccoli in a pan with a few inches of water in it and simmer, covered, until the broccoli turns bright green. *Do not overcook!*
3. Strain water from broccoli if a steamer was not used.
4. Add all of the ingredients to the Vitamix and, starting at 1, turn the dial all the way up to 10. Then put it on High for 2-3 minutes until smooth.
5. Pour it up and serve it immediately. It should be warm at this point from the heat of the motor as well as the heat from the ingredients.
(It's still basically raw.)

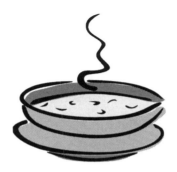

Cauliflower Soup
Makes 2 cups

1 cup raw milk of your choice, warmed but not hot
⅓ cup raw organic cheddar cheese
1 cup cauliflower, barely steamed
¼ cup onion

1. Heat milk gently on the stove, enough to warm it but not kill the enzymes.
2. Steam cauliflower in a steamer (*metal piece designed to go into a pan with a few inches of water underneath it*). If you don't have one, put the cauliflower in a pan with a few inches of water in it and simmer. Do not overcook!
3. Strain water from cauliflower if a steamer was not used.
4. Add all of the ingredients to the Vitamix and, starting at 1, turn the dial all the way up to 10. Then put it on High for a bit until smooth.
5. Pour it up and serve immediately. It should be warm at this point from the heat of the motor as well as the heat from the ingredients.
(It's still basically raw.)

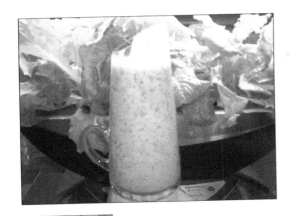

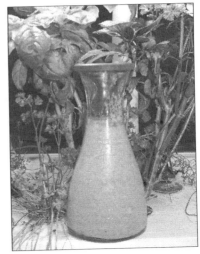

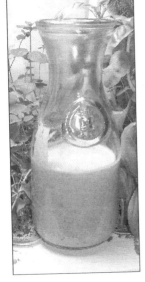

Salad
Dressings

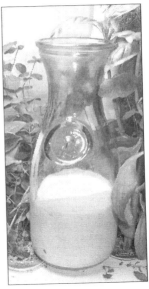

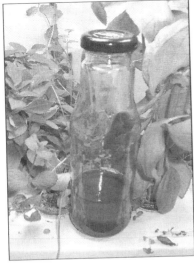

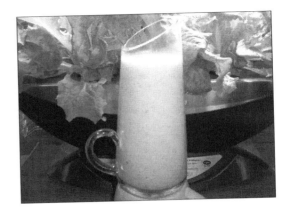

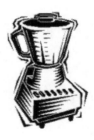

Salad Dressings

One of the easiest things you can do for yourself is to keep a good salad dressing on hand at all times. Then you can just come in, grab some veggies and a dressing, and sit down to a good meal. It doesn't even have to be what most people think of as a salad, that is, lettuce and tomatoes. If you are running through the grocery store and need something fast, think of packaged veggies such as broccoli slaw or carrot slaw.

Granted, it would be much less expensive to buy the veggies, and clean and cut them up yourself. But if you are time crunched, the packages of vegetables that most stores have available these days are a real time saver. Check them out some time when you are not in a hurry so that you know what is available.

I have given you six different salad dressings here that match what most people like to eat. They are fairly easy to make, and I think they taste delicious. In a pinch, you can use EVOO (Extra Virgin Olive Oil), a squeeze of lemon and some sea salt as an easy dressing for a lettuce salad. Check out the Marinated Greens and Marinated Kale in the next section for those dressing recipes.

As long as you have a dressing and some kind of vegetable in your house, preferably from your own garden, you're good to go. Get creative and find unique ways to use different vegetables and pair them with dressings.

Green Goddess Dressing
Makes 6 servings

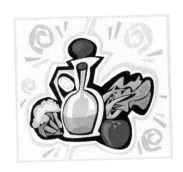 ½ cup lemon juice
1 cup macadamia nuts, soaked for 8 hours and drained
3 cloves garlic, chopped fine
¼ sweet onion
4 stalks of celery
2 teaspoons sea salt
1 teaspoon freshly ground pepper
1 tablespoon fresh parsley
1 teaspoon fresh thyme
1 cup filtered water
1 Medjool or Deglet date, pitted
½ cup Grape Seed oil

1. Place all ingredients, except for the oil, in a blender and blend well.
2. Slowly add the Grape Seed oil and blend to a creamy consistency.
3. Serve at once.

Indicates something that has to be done ahead of time

Salad Dressings

Creamy Italian Dressing
Makes 4 cups

⅓ cup lemon juice
¾ cup extra virgin olive oil
5 cloves garlic
½ teaspoon sea salt
🕐 3 dates soaked in 1 cup filtered water 1-2 hours (reserve water)
⅛ cup fresh oregano
⅛ cup fresh basil
2 teaspoons fresh thyme
2 teaspoons ground Salba or chia seeds

1. Place the lemon juice, oil, garlic, salt, and dates with their water in a blender and blend well.
2. Add oregano, basil and thyme, pulsing only enough to chop the herbs.
3. Add the ground Salba or chia.
4. Pour into a container and serve.

🕐 *Indicates something that needs to be done ahead of time*

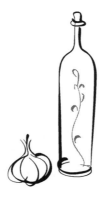

Sesame Miso Dressing
Makes about 1 cup

Miso is a fermented soybean paste commonly used in Asian-style meals. It contains zinc, manganese, copper and Vitamin B12. Fermented soy is the only kind of soy that is good for you to use.

3 tablespoons white miso
3 tablespoons white or brown rice vinegar
A pinch of Stevia
2 teaspoons spicy toasted sesame oil
⅓ cup fresh orange juice
¼ cup plain (not toasted) sesame oil or vegetable oil
1 tablespoon onion, minced

1. In a 2-cup measuring cup, whisk together the miso, vinegar, Stevia and toasted sesame oil until smooth.
2. Whisk in the orange juice.
3. In a steady stream, slowly whisk in the sesame oil until smooth.
4. Stir in the minced onion, and serve on your choice of salad.

This dressing works great on broccoli or cabbage slaw, available pre-made in the produce section of most grocery stores, as well as on green lettuce salads.

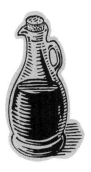

Salad Dressings

Thousand Island Dressing

Makes about 1 cup

½ cup homemade mayonnaise (recipe page 130) or Grapeseed Oil Vegenaise® *(Only use "Follow Your Heart" brand Grapeseed Oil Vegenaise®. It is non-GMO and non-dairy.)*

2 tablespoons Individual Ketchup (see recipe page 132)

¼ cup green or black olives, chopped fine

¼ cup water

⅛ teaspoon paprika

⅛ teaspoon salt

⅛ teaspoon pepper

1. Mix all ingredients together in a bowl.
2. Store in an airtight container in the refrigerator.
3. It will remain soft and spreadable even when chilled.

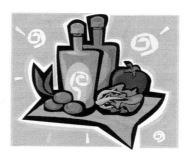

Ranch Dressing

Makes 2 cups

1 cup mayonnaise (see recipe) or Grapeseed Oil Vegenaise®
   (Only use the "Follow Your Heart" brand Grapeseed Oil
Vegenaise®. It's non-GMO and non-dairy.)
1 cup raw milk of your choice (cow, goat, almond, rice, etc.)
¼ teaspoon garlic powder
1 tablespoon onion, diced
1 tablespoon parsley flakes or 2 tablespoons fresh parsley
½ teaspoon black pepper
½ teaspoon sea salt
¾ teaspoon onion powder

1. Combine ingredients in order and stir until smooth.
2. Serve over salad of your choice.
3. Use within two weeks.

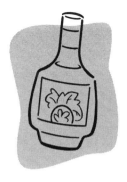

Honey Mustard Dressing
Makes about ½ cup

2 tablespoons balsamic vinegar
1 tablespoon raw honey
1 teaspoon Dijon mustard
¼ teaspoon black pepper
¼ cup olive oil

1. Whisk together all but the olive oil.
2. Slowly add the oil while continuing to whisk to combine it all.
3. Refrigerate until ready to use.

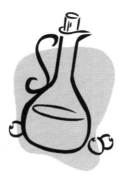

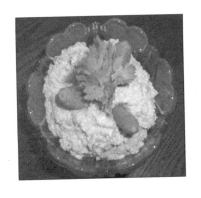

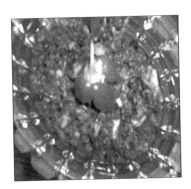

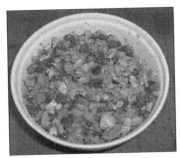

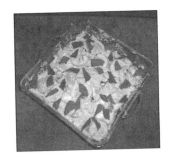

Side
Dishes

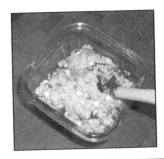

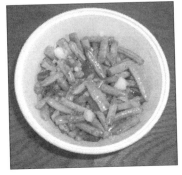

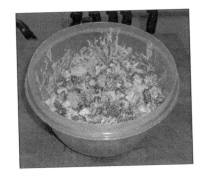

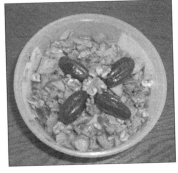

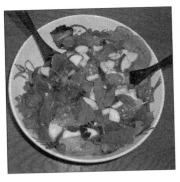

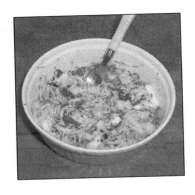

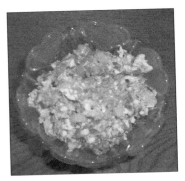

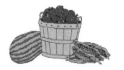

Side Dishes

This section has by far the largest number of recipes, because these are the focus of the book. If you eat two of these side dishes a day with a meat, you will easily reach the goal of eating 5-9 servings of fruits and vegetables daily. In fact, you won't even have to think about it.

Each of these recipes will make around four 16-ounce servings of vegetables (some more, some less). They can go into portable containers, preferably glass, to take with you to work or school. Then when you get home at night, all you have to do is take another one out of the refrigerator and you have dinner for that evening. It doesn't get any simpler than that.

Because I know that holidays happen throughout the year, and that they are notorious for derailing even the best laid plans, I have included recipes for casseroles that serve a crowd, too. Most of these are raw but a few are cooked.

For instance, for Thanksgiving, you could serve Sweetpotato Casserole, Cranberry Salad, Green Beans Almandine, Cranberry Walnut bread, and Raw Pumpkin Pie for dessert. People will want to come back to your house for more, next year, when they taste how good everything is!

Or how about Broccoli with Quick Hollandaise Sauce, Mashed "Faux"-tatoes, Squash Casserole, Marinated Greens, and Zucchini Brownies for dessert? People might start calling you a Gourmet Chef!

I have also included recipes for Marinated Kale and Marinated Chard, and I want you to promise me that you will try them. I could never eat either of these vegetables because they were way too bitter, but I finally found a way to do so, and actually, the kale is my absolute favorite now. I probably eat it every week at some point. And each time I take it to a potluck, people ask me if I will leave them the few leftovers that exist.

The Heavenly Hummus or the Guacamole, served with carrots and celery for dipping, could be used as an appetizer for a party. The possibilities are enormous. So I encourage you to branch out and try things that you might not normally be inclined to make. You just may find that you like something new.

Heavenly Hummus
Makes four 8-ounce servings

🕐   **1 cup soaked garbanzo beans (soak 1 cup chickpeas for 8 hours)**
4 cloves garlic
1 teaspoon cumin powder
1 teaspoon crushed red pepper flakes (optional)
1 teaspoon sea salt
3 tablespoons miso
3 tablespoons tahini
⅓ cup lemon juice
½ cup olive oil

1. Put garlic in food processor and chop.
2. Add soaked garbanzo beans and process.
3. Add cumin, red pepper flakes, and salt, and blend well.
4. Add miso and tahini, and blend.
5. Add lemon juice and oil, and blend until smooth.

Note: Use chickpea miso, found in the refrigerator section of big health food stores, and sometimes even in your local grocery. If unavailable, use white or brown soy miso. Use organic, raw (not roasted) tahini—Maranatha™ brand is a good one. Stir the tahini with a knife before using, to mix in the oil that stays at the top. For olive oil use Extra Virgin Cold Pressed organic.

This should optimally be eaten with raw vegetables such as carrots, celery, broccoli, etc., but may be eaten with flaxseed crackers or homemade chips. Letting it marinate overnight in the refrigerator improves the flavor.

🕐 *Indicates something that needs to be done ahead of time*

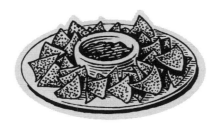

Side Dishes

Marinated Kale

Makes around six 16-ounce servings

2 bunches of kale (or 1 bag of cut up, ready to eat kale)
6 cloves garlic
🕐 **1 Vidalia or sweet onion (Put in freezer for 10 minutes before cutting)**
⅔ cup lemon juice
⅓ cup olive oil
1 teaspoon sea salt

1. Chop kale in a food processor, then put in a large bowl.
2. Add garlic to the processor and chop.
3. Add onion and process with the garlic.
4. Add this to the bowl of chopped kale, and mix thoroughly.
5. Pour lemon juice and olive oil into a measuring cup.
6. Add salt and stir until it dissolves.
7. Pour over the greens like a dressing, stir it in and let it marinate. You can eat it immediately – it does not have to sit overnight.
8. You may add diced red, orange, or yellow bell pepper for holiday color.

If you marinate the kale in a single-serve container, shake it to distribute the dressing before eating. Otherwise, it will just remain at the bottom.

🕐 *Indicates something that needs to be done ahead of time*

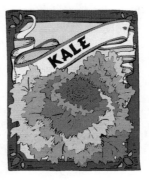

Parsley-Dill Zucchini

Makes two servings

1 large zucchini
2 tablespoons orange or red bell pepper
2 tablespoons chopped onion

Dressing:

½ teaspoon sea salt
¼ cup lemon juice
1 clove garlic
¼ cup olive oil
½ bunch of parsley and/or dill

1. Add salt, lemon juice, garlic and olive oil to blender; blend until smooth.
2. Add the parsley or dill, and pulse the blender until the herbs are chopped.
3. Cut the zucchini up using a Spiral Slicer if you have one, or just chop as you prefer (fine or coarse).
4. Add bell pepper and onion, and stir.
5. Toss dressing with zucchini mixture, stir well, and serve.

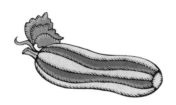

Side Dishes

Carrot Raisin Salad
Serves 8

8-10 carrots
🕐 **1½ cups raisins (soaked 1-2 hours)**
🕐 **½ cup chopped walnuts (soaked overnight and drained)**
Juice of up to 2 lemons (to taste)
Pinch of Stevia

1. Run carrots through food processor, until they are either thin and fine, or big and chunky depending on your liking.
2. Put carrots into a bowl, and add raisins and walnuts.
3. Combine lemon juice and Stevia to make a dressing.
4. Pour over other ingredients in the bowl, and mix.
5. Serve plain, or on lettuce leaves.

🕐 *Indicates something that needs to be done ahead of time*

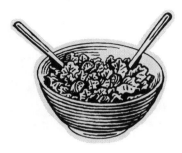

Marinated Greens
Makes 4-5 servings

Three bags of any type greens you like, mixed or all one type.
Assortment of chopped vegetables, preferably organic

Dressing for marinated greens:

1 tablespoon chopped garlic
¼ cup lemon juice
¼ cup Braggs Aminos or Nama Shoyu
½ cup oil (sesame, olive, flax – choose the ones you like the best)
1 tablespoon chopped parsley, or other herbs of your choice

1. Put all greens in a very large bowl. (*I use three bags of organic greens—Spinach, Mixed Baby Greens, Asian Salad Mix, Spring Mix, etc.*)
2. Chop your vegetables of choice (carrots, zucchini, celery, red pepper, etc.) and add them to the greens.
3. Put all the dressing ingredients into a measuring cup and stir.
4. Toss the salad with the dressing until it completely coats all the greens.
5. Put in the refrigerator and let it marinate from 2 to 24 hours. The longer you let it marinate, the better the flavor.

This keeps in the refrigerator for 5-7 days, depending on how fresh the greens are. (*Note: It will seem that three bags of greens plus the vegetables won't fit into the bowl, but this is like a wilted lettuce salad and it will compress greatly as the dressing coats it all.*)

Put in <u>20-ounce</u>, food-grade plastic containers and they're Grab and Go ready!

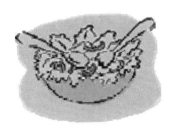

156

Sweetpotato Salad
Makes 4 servings

1 large sweetpotato, peeled
½ cup raisins, soaked 1-2 hours (reserve water)
¼ cup walnuts, soaked 8 hours and chopped into bite-sized pieces
1 tablespoon raisin juice (from soaking water)
½ teaspoon cinnamon, or to taste

1. Chop sweetpotatoes into medium-sized pieces in a food processor.
2. Take potatoes out and put into a serving dish.
3. Drain raisins.
4. Add raisins to sweetpotatoes.
5. Chop walnuts into bite-sized pieces either manually or in the processor, and add to sweetpotatoes.
6. Sprinkle raisin juice over mixture.
7. Sprinkle cinnamon over mixture.
8. Toss well and serve.

Put this into four 16-ounce, food-grade containers for Grab and Go lunches. Glass or ceramic is preferable but plastic can be used since this is not heated.

Indicates something that needs to be done ahead of time

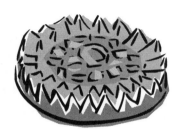

Alive Health Recipe Book

Apple Waldorf Salad
Serves 4-6

4-5 red delicious apples (or whatever kind you prefer), cored and cut into bite-sized pieces in the food processor
2 stalks celery, chopped small
🕐 **¾ cup walnuts, soaked 1-2 hours, drained and chopped small**
🕐 **¾ cup raisins (soaked 1-2 hours)**

Dressing:

½ cup plain yogurt (homemade cow or goat's milk if possible)
A pinch of Stevia to taste
A pinch of sea salt

Alternatively, you can use "Follow Your Heart" brand Grapeseed Oil Vegenaise® as the dressing. Use only Grapeseed—it is non-dairy and non-GMO.

1. Combine the apples, celery, walnuts and raisins.
2. Mix yogurt, salt and Stevia together to make the dressing.
3. Toss, and serve.

The salad should be eaten fairly soon as the apples will turn brown quickly.

🕐 *Indicates something that needs to be done ahead of time*

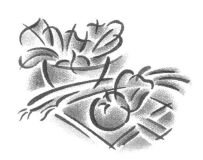

Side Dishes

158

Broccoli Salad

Makes four 8-ounce servings

1 head of broccoli cut into flowerets
🕐 **½ cup of raisins or unsweetened, dried cranberries (soaked 1 - 2 hours)**
🕐 **¼ cup of pine nuts or cashews (soaked 4 hours)**
🕐 **¼ of a purple onion (freeze for 10 minutes before chopping)**
2 stalks celery

Dressing:

1/2 cup yogurt (homemade goat's milk, or coconut milk)
Stevia to taste (if needed)
1 tablespoon of red wine vinegar, to taste

1. Combine the broccoli and next four ingredients in a bowl.
2. Combine dressing ingredients.
3. Pour dressing over salad, and mix thoroughly.

🕐 *Indicates something that needs to be done ahead of time*

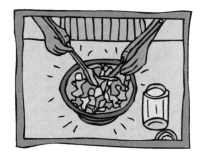

Alive Health Recipe Book

Cranberry Salad
Make about 3 cups

1 pound fresh cranberries (1 bag)
1 naval orange (scrub and use entire orange, including skin, if it is organic; otherwise just use the inside and as much white membrane as possible)
3/4 cup walnuts

1. Cut orange into bite-sized pieces and put into a food processor, along with the cranberries and walnuts.
2. Pulse just a few times so that everything is still in fairly large pieces.
3. Add a little Stevia, to taste.
4. Serve over Romaine lettuce greens or raw spinach.

Goes well with pork, fish, chicken or turkey, and makes a colorful Thanksgiving dish.

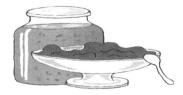

Squash Casserole
Serves 4

Sauce:

🕐 **1 cup pine nuts, soaked 4 hours and drained**
¼ cup unpasteurized white miso
2 cloves garlic
½ teaspoon turmeric
½ cup water
1 tablespoon lemon juice (fresh-squeezed)
1 teaspoon sea salt

Vegetables:

4 yellow or pancake squash, sliced very thin
1 red bell pepper, chopped fine
🕐 **½ large sweet onion, chopped fine (freeze 10 minutes, then chop)**
½ cup spinach, chopped or torn into bite-sized pieces

1. Place sauce ingredients in a blender and blend well; should be thick.
2. Place squash in a bowl and stir in chopped peppers, onions and spinach.
3. Stir sauce into the chopped vegetables.
4. Place in a casserole dish.
5. Place in a dehydrator covered with plastic wrap for 2 hours or more and serve warm, if desired. Dehydrate at 95°. Tastes great warm or cold.

🕐 *Indicates something that needs to be done ahead of time*

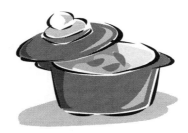

Sweetpotato Casserole
Makes 6 servings

4 cups peeled, chopped sweetpotatoes

½ cup water (from soaking the dates)

🕐 6 dates (soaked 1-2 hours)

1 teaspoon cinnamon

1 teaspoon vanilla extract

🕐 ¼ cup pecans, soaked overnight,* rinsed, and dried on towels

½ cup raisins

Topping:

🕐 ¼ cup pecans, soaked overnight, rinsed and patted dry

1. Puree the chopped sweetpotatoes, water, dates, cinnamon, vanilla, and soaked pecans in a food processor.
2. Pour the mixture into a casserole dish.
3. Fold in the raisins.
4. Scatter the pecan topping over the casserole and serve cold or warmed up.

* Soak ½ cup pecans, then use half in casserole and half for topping

🕐 *Indicates something that needs to be done ahead of time*

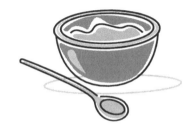

Side Dishes

Tabouli
Makes four 16-ounce servings

2 cloves garlic, minced

2 cups cauliflower florets, chopped very fine to resemble quinoa or bulgur. [*Note: Chop each ingredient separately.*]

🕐 ¾ cup onions, chopped small (put in freezer for 10 minutes first)

¾ cup fresh mint, minced fine

2 stalks celery, chopped fine

1½ cups fresh parsley, minced

3 cups tomatoes, chopped; seed them first
(Brandywines or Romas are best)

Dressing:

¼ cup lemon juice

¼ cup olive oil

1 teaspoon sea salt

1. Place garlic in food processor and chop well to mince.
2. Add cauliflower and chop very fine, then place all of it in a bowl.
3. Process lemon juice, olive oil and salt.
4. Pour this mixture over cauliflower and stir well.
5. Chop the onions, mint, celery, parsley and tomatoes separately.
6. Toss chopped vegetables and herbs together with cauliflower and refrigerate. Shelf Life: 1 week

🕐 *Indicates something that needs to be done ahead of time*

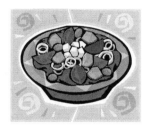

Marinated Chard

Serves 4—Shelf life: 1 week

½ medium onion
1½ cups tomatoes, chopped
2 bunches chard

1. In a food processor, chop the greens first and transfer them to a bowl.
2. Process the onion and tomatoes coarsely and add them to the greens.

Dressing:

2 cloves garlic
1 teaspoon cumin
⅛ cup fresh basil
1 tablespoon oregano
2 teaspoons thyme
¼ cup extra virgin olive oil
1 lime, juiced
1 teaspoon sea salt

1. Place garlic in the food processor and chop fine.
2. Add cumin, oregano, basil and thyme; chop fine.
3. Add olive oil, lime juice and salt.
4. Pour dressing over salad, and massage well until the greens become soft.

Marinate for an hour and serve immediately.

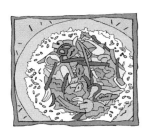

Mashed "Faux"tatoes
Serves 4

1 head of cauliflower
2 tablespoons organic butter (preferably not pasteurized)
¼ teaspoon sea salt
Black pepper to taste
Some raw organic cheddar cheese to go on top (optional)
Chives (optional)

1. Lightly steam the cauliflower over medium heat until tender, or cook in a small amount of water in a saucepan (about 15 minutes).
2. In a food processor or Vitamix, blend cauliflower, butter, sea salt and pepper until smooth.
3. Transfer to a serving bowl, sprinkle with cheese and chives, if desired, and serve immediately.

You'll be surprised by how close these taste to the real thing. (If you don't tell your family, they may not know the difference!)

You can also use either the white gravy or mushroom gravy (see recipes) on top of these for added taste, instead of the cheese and chives.

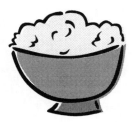

Curried Corn

Serves 2-4

2 cups organic corn (fresh, or one 12 oz. bag of frozen, thawed)
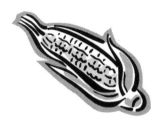 ¼ cup macadamia nuts (soaked 4 hours)
½ teaspoon sea salt
¼ teaspoon ground cumin
2 teaspoons curry powder
½ teaspoon Salba or chia seeds
⅛ teaspoon turmeric
½ small onion, chopped fine (freeze for 10 minutes, then chop)
½ red bell pepper, chopped fine
1 stalk of organic celery, chopped fine

1. Place the corn, soaked nuts, salt, pepper, cumin, curry and turmeric in a blender or food processor and blend until smooth.
2. Add Salba or chia seeds and blend well. If too thick, add filtered water.
3. Add the chopped onion, celery and red pepper; stir to mix.
4. Place in a bowl and serve.

Plan to eat this fairly soon as it does not keep well.

🕐 *Indicates something that needs to be done ahead of time*

Raw Slaw
Makes four 8-ounce servings

1½ cups raw celery, chopped
1½ cups raw cauliflower, chopped
1 cup carrots, shredded
Handful of fresh cilantro, chopped (optional)
½ cup raw, organic, grass-fed cream or yogurt (If using yogurt, add Stevia or Lo Han to taste, just enough to get tartness out)
½ teaspoon prepared ground mustard (in the spice section)

1. Place chopped vegetables in a bowl along with the cilantro.
2. Add mustard to the raw cream or yogurt.
3. Pour dressing over salad.
4. Stir ingredients well to combine.

.

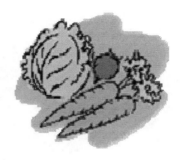

Deli Cole Slaw
(The super easy way)

1 16-ounce package of 3-color Deli Cole Slaw (Fresh Express is one brand; green cabbage, carrots, and red cabbage, or your preference)
1 orange (wedged and halved) **or pineapple** (cut into bite-sized pieces)
½ cup almonds, walnuts, pecans or macadamia nuts

1. Put Cole Slaw into a large bowl.
2. Cut orange or pineapple into pieces and add to Cole Slaw.
3. Add the chopped nuts and stir thoroughly to blend.

Classic Deli Cole Slaw Dressing

½ cup mayonnaise (see note below)
2 tablespoons apple cider vinegar
Dash of Stevia or Lo Han

1. Combine all ingredients.
2. Pour dressing over Cole Slaw, mix well, and serve immediately. Enjoy!

Note: *For the mayonnaise, you can make your own following the recipe in this book, or you can buy "Follow Your Heart" brand Vegenaise® made with Grapeseed oil ONLY. It is sometimes hard to find because it sells out quickly, but my local Kroger carries it in the Nature's Market section, in the dairy case. That's the only kind I recommend buying.*

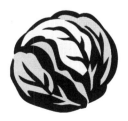

Side Dishes

Colorful Cabbage Salad
Makes three to four 16-ounce Servings

Package of Fresh Express® brand America's Fresh Cole Slaw
⅔ cup parsley, chopped
1 medium scallion, chopped
2 tablespoons grapeseed oil
2 tablespoons apple cider vinegar
1 teaspoon dill weed
1 teaspoon Spike vegetable seasoning or Mrs. Dash
Handful of sunflower seeds, shelled

1. In a large serving bowl, combine cabbage, carrots, parsley and scallion.
2. In a separate bowl, combine oil, vinegar, dill and vegetable seasoning.
3. Pour over salad.
4. Sprinkle sunflower seeds over the top.
5. Refrigerate for at least 20 minutes before serving to improve flavor.

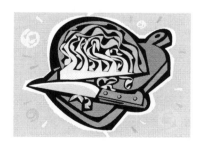

Spinach Mushroom Salad
Makes 1 serving

Handful of spinach, torn into bite-sized pieces
½ cup of mushrooms, cut into bite-sized pieces
1 ounce of raw cheddar or Wisconsin Jack cheese
  (Organic Valley is one brand), cubed
3 ounces of cooked turkey ham (Wilshire Farms), cubed
Extra virgin olive oil
Apple cider vinegar, if desired

1. Arrange spinach on plate.
2. Add mushrooms, cheese, and turkey ham.
3. Drizzle with olive oil as a dressing.
4. Add a bit of apple cider vinegar, if you can tolerate vinegar.

Wilshire Farms turkey ham is a preformed batch of dark turkey meat. It does have a small amount of sugar as one of the ingredients, but it is last on the list. It's so much easier to use and is the only dark turkey or chicken meat that I have found outside of buying a whole bird and cutting it up yourself.

Sweet Rainbow Crunch

Makes approximately four 16-ounce Servings

1 cup purple cabbage
1 cup grated carrots
1 cup chopped celery
1 cup chopped yellow squash
1 cup chopped broccoli
1 cup chopped red bell pepper
1 cup blueberries

Dressing:

⅓ cup lemon juice
¾ cup extra virgin olive oil
5 cloves garlic
½ teaspoon sea salt
🕐 **3 dates soaked in 1 cup filtered water 1-2 hours (reserve water and add to dressing)**
🕐 **½ cup macadamia nuts, soaked overnight**

1. Chop all vegetables singly in food processor and put together in a bowl.
2. Add blueberries and mix thoroughly.
3. Blend lemon juice, oil, garlic, salt, and dates (with water) in a blender.
4. Add in soaked macadamia nuts and blend until smooth.
5. Toss dressing with the salad and let it marinate about 15 minutes.

🕐 *Indicates something that needs to be done ahead of time*

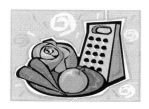

Wild Rice
Makes about 6 servings

This is one example of a "grain" that you can readily eat because it is not a grain at all. It is actually a grass, most of which is also cultivated rather than wild, so it is a complete misnomer.

It is an annual aquatic seed *Zizania aquatica* found mostly in the upper freshwater lakes of Canada, Michigan, Wisconsin, and Minnesota in North America. For an occasional treat, try cooking up this nutty flavored grass with some mushrooms thrown in at the end.

1 package of regular Wild Rice, Paddy Grown

1. In a medium saucepan, bring 2½ cups water and ¼ teaspoon salt to a boil.
2. Stir in the rice, reduce heat, cover, and simmer for about 60 minutes.
3. For firmer texture, decrease cooking time.
4. For softer, more tender texture, increase the cooking time.
5. Once desired texture has been reached, remove from heat.
6. Drain excess liquid, fluff with a fork and serve.

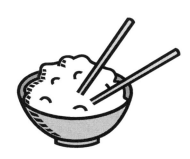

Green Beans Almandine

Serves 6-8

4 cups fresh green beans, cut into bite-sized pieces
1 cup almonds, soaked 8 hrs and drained (you can buy pre-sliced)
2 tablespoons extra virgin olive oil
2 tablespoons lemon juice
1 teaspoon garlic
4 tablespoons onion, chopped
4 tablespoons red bell pepper, chopped
½ teaspoon sea salt
4 teaspoons dried dill or 2 tablespoons fresh (you can use parsley in place of dill)

1. Slice the soaked almonds in a food processor, if purchased whole.
2. Add to green beans.
3. Mix the olive oil, lemon juice, garlic, onion, red bell pepper, sea salt, and dill or parsley together, and pour over beans.
4. Let marinate or serve immediately.

Indicates something that has to be done ahead of time

(Note: There are eight cups in a 32-ounce package of pre-washed green beans if you prefer to buy them that way.)

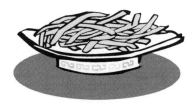

Snap Pea Delight
Serves 8

    1 cup carrots, shredded
    1 cup sugar snap or snow peas
    1 cup chopped tomatoes
    ½ cup extra virgin olive oil
    ½ cup fresh-squeezed orange juice
🕐   **1 cup sunflower seeds (soaked 4 hours in water and drained)**

1. Shred carrots with a grater and put into a medium-sized bowl.
2. Cut peas into bite-sized pieces and add to carrots.
3. Chop tomatoes and add to the bowl.
4. Squeeze the orange for the juice.
5. Mix olive oil with orange juice and pour over ingredients bowl.
6. Add soaked sunflower seeds and mix thoroughly.
7. Marinate for at least two hours before serving.

🕐 *Indicates something that needs to be done ahead of time*

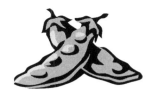

Broccoli with Easy Hollandaise Sauce

Makes about 1 cup of sauce

½ cup butter
2 egg yolks (test eggs first, see page 71)
2 tablespoons lemon juice
½ teaspoon prepared mustard
Dash of white pepper
¼ teaspoon sea salt

1. Heat butter until bubbly but not browned.
2. Put other ingredients in blender and mix well.
3. Add butter *slowly,* and continue to mix until thick and creamy.
4. Pour into a serving dish and serve over broccoli.

Steamed Broccoli

1. Put a steamer into a saucepan and turn heat on.
2. Place broccoli in steamer and cover with lid.
3. Let the broccoli steam lightly until it turns bright green.
4. Remove from steamer, pour sauce over broccoli, and serve immediately.

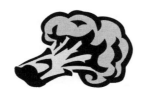

Guacamole
Makes 4 Servings

4 avocados
¼ sweet Vidalia onion
2 cloves garlic
1 teaspoon sea salt
1 lime, juiced
1 teaspoon cumin
1 teaspoon fresh cilantro
3 stalks celery
1 small tomato

1. Place garlic in food processor and chop fine.
2. Add onion and process.
3. Add avocados, lime juice, salt, cumin, and cilantro, and process.
4. Take out and put into a bowl.
5. Dice tomato and celery and add to bowl.
6. Serve over Portobello mushrooms for a hearty meal, or with homemade chips or crackers for an appetizer.

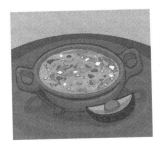

Side Dishes

Zucchini Alfredo

Makes about 6 servings

4-5 zucchinis, depending on size
Paprika for garnish

Alfredo Sauce:

½ cup butter
1 eight-ounce package of cream cheese
2 teaspoons garlic powder
2 cups raw milk
6 ounces grated parmesan cheese
⅛ teaspoon black pepper
¼ cup fresh parsley, chopped

1. Use Saladacco or spiral slicer to cut zucchini into "noodles."
2. Melt butter in a saucepan over medium heat.
3. Add the cream cheese, and garlic powder, and whisk until smooth.
4. Add the milk slowly, and whisk to smooth out any lumps.
5. Add parmesan and pepper and stir desired consistency is reached.
6. Stir in parsley, and serve over "noodles."
7. Optionally, add chicken to turn it into an entree.

If the sauce cooks too long or becomes thick, thin with more milk.

I know this recipe is cooked, and much of the dairy is pasteurized, but every so often you can splurge. This is divinely decadent, so I decided to add it in.

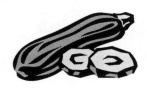

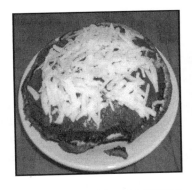
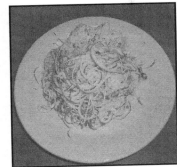
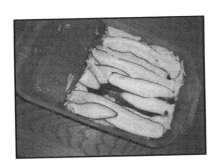
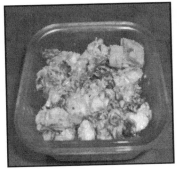

Main
Meals

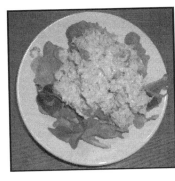
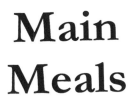
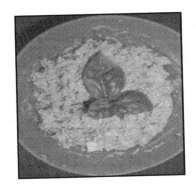
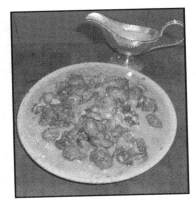
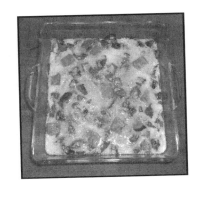
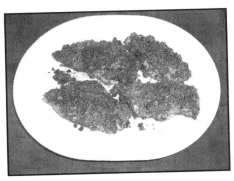
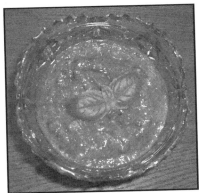

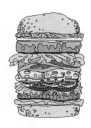

Main Meals

I called this section Main Meals because the word Entrees didn't really fit it very well. If you have read Part One, you will understand what I use for meat most of the time. These are just examples of other things that you can use. Remember, the whole idea of this book is to prepare quick, simple meals for on-the-go eating.

Plus, I know there will be times when special occasions arise, or when you may be having people over for dinner on holidays. I have included some more time-consuming (but really tasty) dishes to prepare for those events. The Chia Chicken and the Swedish Meatballs are two examples of special dishes that are still wheat-free, gluten-free, sugar-free and artificial sweetener-free. They happen to both be dairy-free too, if that is important to you.

The Spinach Mushroom bake is a great brunch dish to serve guests, and the Spaghetti and Lasagna are nice enough to be fancy dishes, as well. Besides being delicious, they are certainly different, and will be conversation pieces.

Please read the chapters on coconut oil and natural sweeteners if you haven't already done so. Then you will understand why I use them, and how wonderfully good they are for you.

The rest of the recipes are just good old-fashioned stand-bys with a twist—they are all healthy and good for you. Hopefully, they will give you the inspiration to adapt some of your own favorite recipes, as well as to try different combinations of dishes from various sections of this book. Healthy eating to you!

Tomato Basil Sauce

Recipe makes enough for four 16-oz. servings of spaghetti, 1 large lasagna and 4 pizzas

4 cloves garlic
🕐 **9 dates (soaked 1-2 hours)**
🕐 **3 cups sun-dried tomatoes (soaked 1-2 hours)**
🕐 **Half of a sweet onion (put in freezer 10 min. before chopping)**
1 teaspoon fresh oregano
1 teaspoon fresh thyme
1½ cups fresh basil
6 cups fresh tomatoes
3 tablespoons lemon juice
1 teaspoon sea salt
3 tablespoons olive oil

1. Put garlic in the food processor and chop.
2. Add dates and blend well (*check that there are no pits in the dates*).
3. Add sun-dried tomatoes and blend.
4. Then add rest of the ingredients and blend until smooth.
5. Put in refrigerator and let sit overnight so that the flavors meld.
6. Use strips of zucchini as "spaghetti" to put the sauce over. If you have a Saladacco cutter, it will spiral cut the zucchini so that it looks like spaghetti. (Spaghetti squash works well, too.)

This is great served cold in the summer, or you can gently heat it on the stove in a double boiler, to warm it up for colder months. (This still keeps the enzymes and nutrients alive.)

🕐 *Indicates something that needs to be done ahead of time*

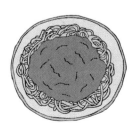

"Spaghetti"

Healthy spaghetti is made from **all the left-over zucchini** that you have in your garden (or your neighbors have in theirs). It is amazing how wonderful it tastes, while still being good for you.

Zucchini "noodles" are used with the spaghetti sauce (see previous page) or with the Zucchini Alfredo which is found on page 176. To make this spaghetti, you will need a Saladacco, which is fairly easy to find, or a Spirooli, which is a bit more difficult to locate (see the Resources Section for information on where to find both).

To make the spaghetti, cut the washed zucchini into sections about three inches long. Then put each section under the top part of the Saladacco with the blade control turned to the left for slicing. Turning it to the right will make scallops.

Lock the top closed and start turning the handle. You will see the "noodles" come out of the bottom into the holding container. When you have done all the sections of zucchini, you can choose what sauce you want to put over it.

There are three here to choose from: the mushroom sauce, the tomato sauce or the cheese (Alfredo) sauce. Try them all and see which one is your favorite!

[If you prefer, spaghetti squash "noodles" may be used with these sauces, instead.]

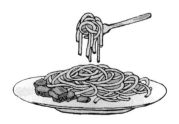

Lasagna
Serves 6-8 people

Tomato Basil Sauce (see page 179)
1-2 zucchinis, depending on size
Parmesan cheese, grated
Provolone cheese, grated (may substitute raw cheddar cheese)
Meat of your choice: salmon or chicken sausage, ground beef, chicken, or turkey (preferably organic and free-range)

1. Prepare the meat to your liking, using a small amount of coconut oil in a frying pan. Just heat the sausage through or brown the other meat.
2. Add the meat to the tomato basil sauce and *gently* heat it, or use it cold.
3. Cut the zucchinis in thin strips lengthwise using a V-slicer or cheese slicer, and layer the bottom of a casserole dish with them.
4. Add a layer of meat sauce, and then the grated Provolone cheese.
5. Repeat the layering once more, ending with a layer of zucchini.
6. Sprinkle the grated Parmesan cheese on top and heat in the dehydrator for three hours at 95° to serve it warm. Otherwise you may eat it cold.

Note: Provolone and Parmesan cheeses are both naturally low in lactose and are therefore good choices for this dish.

Main Meals

Chilled Chicken Curry Salad
Makes 3-4 Servings

1½ cups light and dark meat chicken, cooked and chopped
1 cup chopped Granny Smith apples (or fresh cranberries)
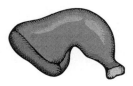 ½ cup raw almonds, soaked for 8 hours and sliced
1 tablespoon parsley
1 stalk celery
½ to ¾ cup fresh, raw cream, or yogurt (preferably homemade)
Dash of Stevia or Lo Han, to taste
½ rounded teaspoon curry paste or curry powder, to taste

1. Place chicken, apples, almonds, parsley, and celery into medium-sized bowl.
2. Measure out raw cream or yogurt, and add sweetener and curry.
5. Pour curry mixture over chicken, and stir well to combine.
6. Serve cold over lettuce or spinach.

Indicates something that needs to be done ahead of time

Chia Chicken

Serves 4

Chicken—4 boneless, skinless breasts or thighs
2 tablespoons ground chia seeds
  (grind in a coffee grinder dedicated to this purpose)
⅓ cup almond meal
1 tablespoon olive oil
1 tablespoon almond butter
1 teaspoon lemon juice
1 teaspoon sea salt
Pinch cayenne pepper
1 teaspoon fresh parsley
¼ teaspoon paprika
1 teaspoon fresh thyme
1 tablespoon onion, finely chopped

1. Preheat oven to 350°F.
2. If chicken pieces are not even, pound them flat using a kitchen mallet.
3. In a flat dish or plate, mix together olive oil, almond butter, lemon juice, onions, spices, and herbs.
4. Coat chicken with mixture. Time permitting, marinate for 10-15 minutes.
5. Remove chicken and place on baking sheet covered with parchment paper.
6. Pour almond meal and ground chia into small bowl and stir to mix evenly.
7. Coat chicken on both sides with almond/chia mixture, patting with hands to better adhere the "crust" to the chicken.
8. Place baking sheet in center of oven and bake for 20-30 minutes, or until an instant read thermometer reaches 168° on the thickest part.

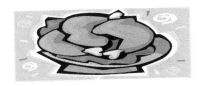

Main Meals

Tuna Salad
Serves one

1 3.75 ounce can of low mercury tuna (Vital Choice)
1 tablespoon of homemade mayonnaise (see recipe)
1 stalk of celery, cut into bite-sized pieces
1 tablespoon of onion (optional)

1. Put tuna fish into a small bowl.
2. Add other ingredients to taste.
3. Serve over a bed of romaine lettuce (and eat the lettuce too!)

You can put the tuna fish plain into a larger mixed salad for extra protein. Vital Choice has excellent, third-party certified pure, dolphin safe tuna that can be ordered through their catalog or on the internet.

Alternatively, you can use "Follow Your Heart" brand Vegenaise® made with Grapeseed oil ONLY for the mayonnaise. It is sometimes hard to find because it sells out quickly, but my local Kroger carries it in the Nature's Market section in the dairy case. You can also get it at organic stores. That's the only kind I recommend buying.

Variations on this recipe are endless. You can add a chopped boiled egg, some chopped apple, pickle relish (remember, it has sugar, so just a little) or additional fruits and vegetables.

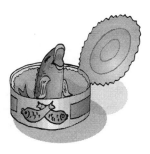

Salmon Salad
Serves one

1 7.5 ounce can *Vital Choice* **Wild Red Alaskan sockeye salmon**
2 tablespoons homemade mayonnaise (see recipe) or Veganaise®
1 Individual Serving of Ketchup (optional—see recipe below)
1 teaspoon horseradish sauce (optional)
1 tablespoon chopped onion
1 stalk of celery, chopped

1. Put salmon, with its oil, in a small bowl.
2. Add mayonnaise to taste.
3. Mix in the individual serving of ketchup (double it, if preferred).
4. Add the horseradish sauce to taste (optional).
5. Stir in chopped onion and celery.
6. Mix well and serve over lettuce leaves or eat as is.

Individual Serving of Ketchup

1 tablespoon organic tomato puree or tomato paste
¾ teaspoon apple cider vinegar
Pinch of Stevia, to taste
¼ teaspoon garlic, finely minced
¼ teaspoon basil, minced

Whisk all ingredients together in a small bowl. Double or triple the amount as your recipe calls for ketchup. This is a sugar-free recipe that you can make up in small amounts since there are no preservatives in it.

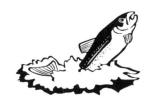

Main Meals

Swedish Meatballs
Serves 4-6

Mushroom Gravy (see recipe on page 135)
1 pound of grass-fed, grass-finished ground beef
Salt and pepper to taste
2 tablespoons of coconut oil
2 zucchini squash

1. Make the mushroom gravy according to the recipe.
2. Add salt and pepper to the ground beef and shape it into balls.
3. Sauté meatballs in coconut oil until cooked medium rare. Do not overcook, or the meat will be tough.
4. Add meatballs to mushroom gravy at the end of cooking.
5. Use a Saladacco to cut zucchini into "spaghetti" noodles or chop them up.
6. Mix noodles into the gravy and meatballs, just to warm them.
7. Serve on individual plates.

If there are any leftovers, refrigerate them, and when ready to eat again, gently heat everything in a pan on the stove, barely enough to warm it up.

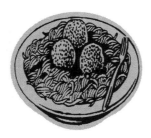

Personal Raw Pizza
Serves One

1 Portobello mushroom per person
Tomato Sauce (see recipe on page 179)
Grated raw organic cheddar cheese (Organic Valley, etc.)
Toppings of your choice

1. Take center stem out of mushroom. Chop stem to use for topping.
2. Turn the mushroom over, and spread tomato sauce inside the cap.
3. Put whatever amount of cheese you like on top of the sauce.
4. Add the toppings of your choice, including the chopped mushroom stem.
5. Enjoy!

A Portobello mushroom has a lot of protein in it and will fill you up pretty quickly. You can always have another one on hand if you want more than one. Toppings can include, but are not limited to, ground beef, chicken or turkey (cooked low and slow in coconut oil on the stove), broccoli, onions, squash, etc. Use your imagination and whatever is on hand in your garden or kitchen.

Alternatively, you can buy a gluten-free pizza crust at many stores. Then make pizza the same way you would using a regular crust.

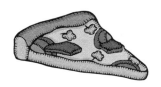

Spinach Mushroom Bake

Makes 9 servings

Handful of spinach, torn into bite-sized pieces
1 cup mushrooms, cut into bite-sized pieces
3 ounces of cooked turkey ham or other meat, chopped
2 ounces of raw cheddar cheese, mild or sharp, grated
6 eggs
¼ cup raw milk of your choice (cow, goat, coconut, etc.)
¼ teaspoon sea salt
Dash of pepper, to taste
½ teaspoon ground prepared mustard (in the spice aisle)
🕐 ¼ stick (2 tablespoons) butter, melted

1. Preheat oven to 350°F.
2. Place torn spinach over the bottom of a greased, square glass baking dish.
3. Spread mushrooms and turkey ham evenly over the spinach.
4. In a medium bowl, break the eggs, and stir gently to mix.
5. To eggs, add the melted butter, milk, mustard, salt, and pepper. Stir.
6. Pour mixture over the spinach and mushrooms.
7. Sprinkle grated cheese over the top.
8. Cover the dish with foil and bake at 350° for 20-25 minutes.

🕐 *Indicates something that needs to be done ahead of time*

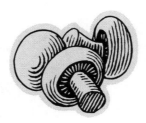

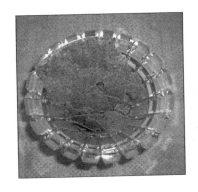
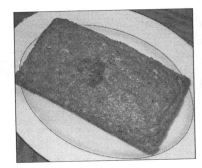
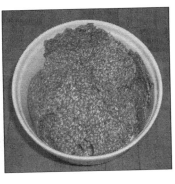
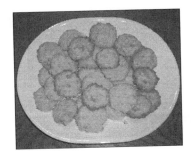

Crackers
And Breads

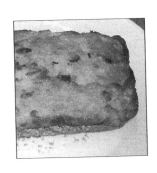
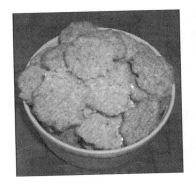
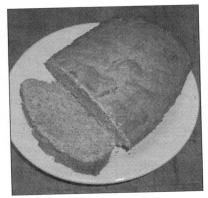
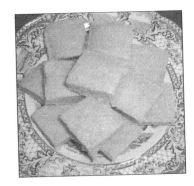
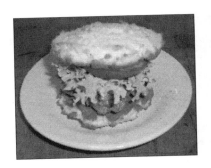
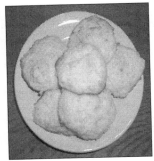
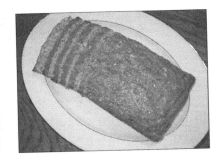

Crackers and Breads

This section has recipes that try to satisfy your cravings for snacks like chips. It also contains a recipe for hamburger buns, should you still desire bread. Personally, I don't miss bread much at all, and prefer to eat my meat by itself. However, I know that people have to go in steps and stages to get to the point of abandoning wheat products.

It is my goal to find something healthy to replace the chips that most people consume, almost without thinking about it. Hopefully, these recipes have met and even exceeded that goal. Most commercial bags of potato chips, for example, have awful ingredients that make you crave them to the point that you literally "can't eat just one." My recipes for homemade chips will not cause such cravings, while still giving you the satisfaction of a snack.

I've been known to wolf down a whole box of crackers, or bag of chips, then notice with amazement that I did so. You probably have had the same, or a similar, experience. The manufacturers put things like MSG (or any of its derivations) in the chips in vast quantities to stimulate your appetite, and make you want more. Read more about it on page 24.

Corn is a grain that is really not good for anyone to eat. Ideally, you should reduce and eventually eliminate all grains from your diet. But if you still crave the taste, the corn chip recipe in this section should give you a good substitute for the chips on store shelves.

Once you have gotten your body accustomed to eating well, and have regained your health, you may find that you no longer have any cravings for these types of things. I don't anymore, but watch out if you ever pick one up at a friend's house or a party. You can quickly become addicted all over again.

All of the bread recipes, again, are wheat-free, gluten-free, sugar-free and artificial sweetener-free, just like other recipes in this book. Coconut oil is used copiously. If you are unfamiliar with it, please read in Chapter 3, page 35 about this incredibly healthy and good-for-you product. Also read about the natural sweeteners on page 55 so that you are familiar with them as well.

Again, the breads can be used either as snacks, or desserts, and are easily transported. So make a double batch, and freeze some for later! That way you'll never be caught short.

Flaxseed Crackers

Makes approximately 6 dozen crackers

⏱ ⅔ cup sun-dried tomatoes (soaked 2 hours and drained)
⏱ 2 cups flaxseeds, ground, and soaked for ½ hour in 3 cups water
2 tablespoons chopped garlic
1 cup fresh cilantro or 3 tablespoons dried
3 teaspoons crushed red pepper flakes (optional)
¾ cup fresh tomatoes
⅓ cup red bell pepper
1 tablespoon olive oil
2 teaspoons sea salt
6 tablespoons Braggs Amino Acids

1. Soak the flaxseeds as above. They will look like jelly. Do not rinse them.
2. Chop the garlic first in the food processor.
3. Chop the cilantro and add the red pepper flakes.
4. Add the tomatoes, process, and then add the sun-dried tomatoes; blend.
5. Process the bell pepper, olive oil, Braggs and sea salt.
6. Put the flaxseed mixture into the food processor and blend well.
7. Spread mixture out thinly onto two Teflex sheets and dehydrate for 24 hours at 90°F. Peel away the Teflex sheet and continue to dehydrate until desired crispness is reached (about 12 more hours).
8. When the crackers are ready, take them out and break into pieces.
9. Store in an airtight container or plastic bags in the refrigerator.

Note: Crackers may be baked in an oven on lowest setting, on parchment-lined cookie sheet.

⏱ *Indicates something that needs to be done ahead of time*

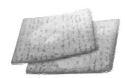

Crackers and Breads

Barbecue Flax Crackers

Makes approximately 3 dozen crackers

🕐 **1 cup golden flaxseeds (soaked overnight)**
1 cup water
½ cup Barbecue Sauce (see recipe on page 131)

1. Soak the flaxseeds in the one cup of water overnight. They will expand, so make sure you have a two-cup capacity for soaking.
2. After soaking, combine the half cup of barbecue sauce with the flaxseeds.
3. Stir to mix thoroughly, and spread thinly over one Teflex dehydrator sheet.
4. Dehydrate at 105°F until done, turning over halfway through.
5. When turning over, remove from Teflex sheet, and continue to dry on the mesh sheet only. Crackers are done when dry all the way around.
6. Once dry, break up into cracker-sized pieces and store in an airtight container in the refrigerator.

Dehydrating time will vary greatly with climate, altitude, humidity, and heat. These should take about 6 to 10 hours to dry.

Note: Crackers may be baked in an oven on lowest setting, on parchment-lined cookie sheet.

🕐 *Indicates something that needs to be done ahead of time*

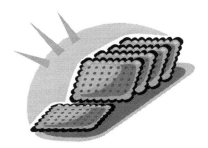

Corn Chips
Makes about 6 dozen chips

🕐 1 cup shelled sunflower seeds, soaked overnight, then rinsed
2½ cups fresh corn, or a 16 oz. bag of frozen organic; thawed
1 teaspoon sea salt
1 teaspoon chili powder
1 teaspoon turmeric
½ cup water
🕐 2 Tbsp. flaxseed, soaked in 4 Tbsp. water, for 15 minutes

1. Combine all except flaxseed in a blender or food processor, and puree.
2. Stir in the flaxseed.
3. Drop the mixture by spoonfuls onto solid Teflex dehydrator sheets in thin, flat, 4-inch rounds. Flatten them with back of spoon if necessary.
4. Dehydrate chips at 105°F until they are crisp on one side.
5. Turn the chips over and continue dehydrating until they are dry on the other side (about 12-15 hours total).

Dehydrating time will vary greatly with climate, altitude, humidity and heat. The times given are approximations.

Note: Chips may be baked in an oven on lowest setting, on parchment-lined cookie sheet.

🕐 *Indicates something that needs to be done ahead of time*

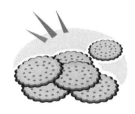

Crackers and Breads

Barbecue Corn Chips
Makes approximately 3 dozen chips

2 cups fresh corn, or a 10 oz. bag frozen organic corn; thawed
½ cup Barbecue Sauce (see recipe on page 131)
Extra water in case the blender starts straining

1. Cut corn off cob, or thaw out frozen corn.
2. Put in a Vitamix blender, or food processor.
3. Add the half cup of barbecue sauce in with corn.
4. Blend until very smooth. Add water as needed to prevent motor strain.
5. Spread on a Teflex sheet evenly to all corners (very thinly).
6. Dehydrate at 105°F to desired crispiness. If you like your chips crisp, dry them for longer. If you like them chewy, cut some time off. (*I happen to like mine kind of chewy.*)
7. Take chips off the Teflex halfway through drying and leave them on the mesh sheet only for the rest of the time.
8. Once completely dry, break into chip-sized pieces, and store in an airtight container in the refrigerator.

These are really yummy and a good substitute if you still crave chips of any kind. However, it is best to limit, with the idea of eventually eliminating, all grains and starches from your diet.

Note: Chips may be baked in an oven on lowest setting, on parchment-lined cookie sheet.

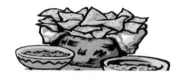

Nacho Corn Chips

Makes approximately 6 dozen chips

2½ cups fresh corn, or 16 oz. bag of frozen organic corn; thawed
1 medium zucchini (six to eight inches long)
2 cloves of garlic
¼ teaspoon sea salt
½ teaspoon cayenne pepper, or more, to taste
⅓ cup flaxseed, ground in dedicated coffee grinder

1. Place all ingredients except flaxseed in food processor and process.
2. Add the ground flaxseed and continue to process until smooth.
3. Spread evenly on a Teflex dehydrator sheet (should be about ⅛" thick).
4. Dehydrate at 105°F for 4-6 hours, depending on desired crispness.
5. Turn chips over and peel off the Teflex sheet after about 2-3 hours.
6. Continue dehydrating chips on the mesh sheet until done.

Dehydrating time will vary greatly with climate, altitude, humidity and heat. The times given are approximations.

Note: Chips may be baked in an oven on lowest setting, on parchment-lined cookie sheet.

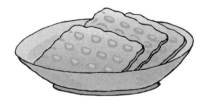

Crackers and Breads

Cheese Drops

Makes about 8 drops

4 eggs
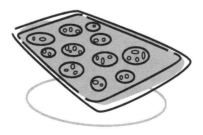 **¼ cup butter or coconut oil, melted**
¼ teaspoon salt
¼ teaspoon onion powder
¼ teaspoon garlic powder
⅓ cup sifted coconut flour
¼ teaspoon baking powder
½ cup raw sharp cheddar cheese (Organic Valley or other), grated

1. Preheat oven to 325°F.
2. Mix together eggs, butter or oil, salt, onion powder, and garlic powder.
3. Combine coconut flour with baking powder and sift into batter.
4. Whisk together until there are no lumps.
5. Fold in cheese.
6. Drop batter by the spoonful onto a cookie sheet, either greased or covered with parchment paper.
7. Bake at 325° for 30 minutes.
8. If you like more cheese, increase the amount to ¾ cup.

Indicates something that needs to be done ahead of time

Cheese Rounds
Makes about 32 rounds

½ cup almond flour
2 eggs
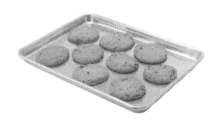 ¼ cup melted butter or coconut oil
¼ teaspoon onion powder
¼ teaspoon sea salt
3 cups organic raw sharp cheddar cheese, shredded
½ cup sifted coconut flour

1. Preheat oven to 325°F.
2. In a bowl, mix together almond flour, eggs, butter or oil, salt, and cheese.
3. Add the coconut flour and knead the dough for 2 to 3 minutes.
4. Form the dough into 1" balls.
5. Place on a cookie sheet covered with parchment paper and flatten to about 2--2½" diameter rounds.
6. Bake at 325° for 30 minutes.

Leftovers can be reheated at 400° for about 4 minutes. They taste best straight from the oven. Almond flour can be purchased, or made by grinding almonds to a fine powder in a Vitamix. (Other nut flours can be made the same way.)

🕐 *Indicates something that needs to be done ahead of time*

Crackers and Breads

Hamburger Buns
Makes 6 buns

      6 eggs
🕐   **½ cup melted butter**
      Pinch of Stevia
      ½ teaspoon sea salt
      ¾ cup sifted coconut flour
      1 teaspoon baking powder

1. Preheat oven to 350°F.
2. In a bowl, mix together eggs, butter, Stevia, and sea salt.
3. Sift coconut flour and baking powder into the bowl.
4. Stir batter until there are no lumps.
5. Pour batter onto a muffin top pan* and bake at 350° for 20 minutes.
6. Remove from pan and cool on a rack before using for hamburgers.

This can be made into a bread and used for sandwiches, too. Pour batter into a greased 9x5x3" or smaller loaf pan, and bake at 350° for 40 minutes. Cool on a rack before cutting.

*Muffin top baking pans may be purchased online at Bob's Red Mill. It's called a 6 Hole Puffy Muffin Crown Pan SKU # 4606-01 for $11.19 at the time of this writing. See "Low and Slow" in Chapter 4 for info on how to cook beef.

🕐 *Indicates something that has to be done ahead of time*

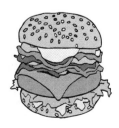

Banana Nut Bread
Makes 1 Loaf

1 cup Xylitol
½ cup melted butter
2 eggs
3 crushed ripe bananas
2 cups oat flour
½ teaspoon sea salt
½ teaspoon baking soda
½ teaspoon aluminum-free baking powder
Splash of apple cider vinegar (this helps it to rise)
½ cup chopped nuts, optional

1. Preheat oven to 350°F.
2. Combine dry ingredients (except nuts) in a small bowl.
3. Cream butter and Xylitol together.
4. Add eggs and apple cider vinegar, and mix well.
5. Stir bananas into bowl, alternating with dry ingredients.
6. Mix until flour disappears.
7. Fold in nuts and pour into a greased loaf pan.
8. Bake at 350° for one hour.
9. Cool on a rack before serving.

Using a piece of parchment paper cut to fit the pan makes clean-up easier. Also, if oat flour is not available, you may grind 2½ cups old-fashioned oats in a Vitamix to make it yourself.

Indicates something that needs to be done ahead of time

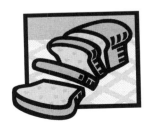

Crackers and Breads

Corn Bread
Makes 8 servings

6 eggs
⏱ **⅓ cup butter or coconut oil, melted**
⅓ cup Xylitol
½ teaspoon vanilla
½ teaspoon salt
¼ cup sifted coconut flour
½ teaspoon baking powder
⅓ cup cornmeal

1. Preheat oven to 400°F.
2. Blend together eggs, butter, Xylitol, vanilla, and salt.
3. Combine coconut flour, baking powder, and cornmeal, and whisk into batter until there are no lumps.
4. Fill greased 8x8x2" baking dish.
5. Bake at 400° for 15-18 minutes.

Use a piece of parchment paper cut to fit the pan for easier clean–up.

⏱ *Indicates something that has to be done ahead of time*

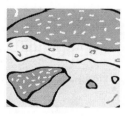

Sweetpotato Bread
Makes 1 Loaf

½ cup cooked sweetpotato
8 eggs
½ cup coconut oil or butter, melted
½ cup Xylitol
1 teaspoon vanilla
1½ teaspoons ground cinnamon
½ teaspoon ground mace
½ teaspoon salt
¾ cup sifted coconut flour
1 teaspoon baking powder
½ cup pecans or walnuts, chopped

1. Preheat oven to 350°F.
2. Cut ½ cup sweetpotato into small chunks. Place in pot with a few inches of water and simmer 15-20 minutes (or use a steamer). Drain and mash.
3. Mix sweetpotato, eggs, oil, Xylitol, vanilla, cinnamon, mace, and salt.
4. Sift coconut flour with baking powder, and whisk thoroughly into batter until there are no lumps.
5. Fold in nuts.
6. Pour into greased 9x5x3" loaf pan and bake at 350° for one hour.
7. Remove from pan and cool on rack.

(Use parchment paper cut to fit the pan for easy clean-up later.) You can use ½ cup canned pumpkin instead, but you will have a lot left over. At least the extra sweetpotato can be used in sweetpotato salad or casserole.

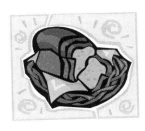

Crackers and Breads

Cranberry Walnut Bread
Makes 1 Loaf

8 eggs
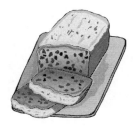 **½ cup coconut oil or butter, melted**
½ cup coconut milk
¾ cup Xylitol (½ cup if using sweetened cranberries)
1 teaspoon vanilla
1 teaspoon lemon extract
½ teaspoon salt
⅔ cup sifted coconut flour
1 teaspoon baking powder
1 cup dried cranberries, unsweetened
½ cup walnuts, chopped

1. Preheat oven to 350°F.
2. Mix eggs, oil, coconut milk, Xylitol, vanilla, lemon extract, and salt.
3. Sift coconut flour with baking powder; whisk thoroughly into batter until there are no lumps.
4. Fold in cranberries and nuts.
5. Pour into greased 9x5x3" loaf pan; bake at 350° for one hour.
6. Remove from pan and cool on rack.

🕐 *Indicates something that has to be done ahead of time*

Zucchini Bread

¾ cup loosely packed, shredded zucchini
8 eggs
½ cup coconut oil or butter, melted
½ cup Xylitol
1 teaspoon vanilla
1½ teaspoons ground cinnamon
½ teaspoon ground mace
½ teaspoon sea salt
¾ cup sifted coconut flour
1 teaspoon baking powder
½ cup pecans or walnuts, chopped

1. Preheat oven to 350°F.
2. Mix the zucchini, eggs, oil, sweetener, vanilla, cinnamon, mace, and salt.
3. Sift coconut flour with baking powder, and whisk thoroughly into batter until there are no lumps.
4. Fold in nuts.
5. Pour into greased 9x5x3" loaf pan; bake at 350° for one hour.
6. Remove from pan and cool on rack before serving.

Use parchment paper cut to fit the pan for easier cleanup and to keep any aluminum or Teflon away from the baked goods, if using one of these pans.

Indicates something that has to be done ahead of time

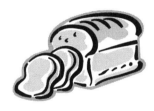

Crackers and Breads

Oatmeal Pumpkin Bread

Makes two loaves and tastes like an oatmeal pumpkin cookie

3 cups oat flour
2 cups Xylitol
½ teaspoon baking soda
1 teaspoon aluminum-free baking powder
½ teaspoon salt
½ teaspoon cinnamon
Splash of apple cider vinegar (this helps it rise)
2 cups cooked pumpkin (or 1 can)
🕐 **1 cup coconut oil, melted**
4 large eggs
1 teaspoon vanilla

1. Preheat oven to 350°F.
2. Mix all of the dry ingredients together in one bowl.
3. Mix all of the wet ingredients together in a separate bowl.
4. Stir dry ingredients into wet ones, mixing thoroughly.
5. Pour into two greased loaf pans.
6. Bake in a 350° oven for one hour, or until done.

If oat flour is not available, grind 3¾ cups old-fashioned (not quick cooking) oatmeal to a fine powder in a Vitamix to make your own.

🕐 *Indicates something that needs to be done ahead of time*

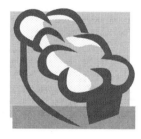

Alive Health Recipe Book

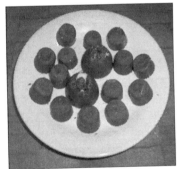
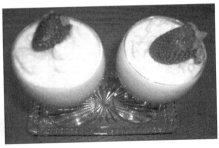
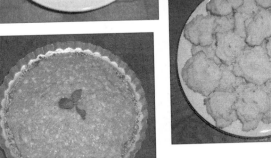
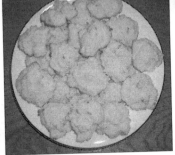
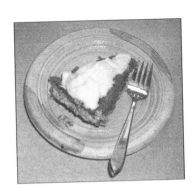

Desserts

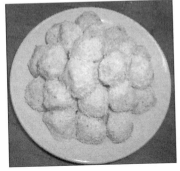
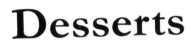
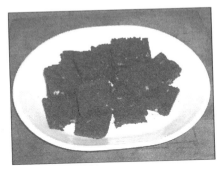
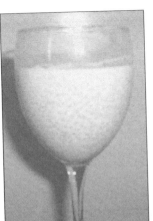
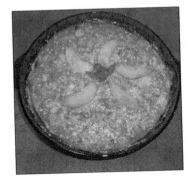
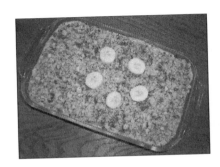
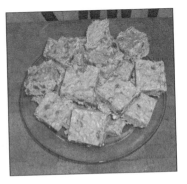

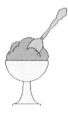

Desserts

These desserts are all wheat-free, gluten-free, sugar-free and artificial sweetener-free. When any one of the recipes calls for milk, it should be raw; not pasteurized or homogenized. Please see Chapter 3, page 40, for the thinking behind this.

You have a choice in the type milk that you use. In the ice cream category, I have one recipe that doesn't use milk at all—the zucchini ice cream. You'll never believe how yummy that one tastes until you try it!

If you choose to go vegan, or non-dairy, you can make your own nut milks per the recipes in Chapter 3, page 52, and substitute that, or buy ready made Rice or Almond milk at the store. But please, NO SOY MILK. Chapter 2, page 27, explains some of the dangers associated with Soy.

Of course, many of these desserts can be used as snacks, too, and most are portable, with the exception of the ice creams. You can use the muffins from the breakfast section for desserts as well, so there should be plenty of choices to end your meal.

Most of these items will freeze well, so you can make up a batch ahead of time and just thaw something out when you need it. That would be a wise use of your time, so you're never caught short and therefore tempted by non-healthy items.

All of the recipes use coconut oil, which, in case you aren't aware of it already, is incredibly good for you. Please see "Good Fats/Bad Fats" in Chapter 3, page 35, for details.

Within the desserts section, there are recipes for candy, cookies, pies, cakes, puddings, brownies and ice cream. Many are very quick to make and can be done at the last minute—try the raw brownies, the chocolate covered strawberries, bananas, etc., plus the ice creams.

Most of the recipes are pretty easy, but I added in a few for any special occasions that may arise. These might require a little bit more effort . The Mango Macadamia pie is one of my favorites, but it does take a bit more time to prepare.

The cake is for special times like birthdays, or holidays. You can frost it with vanilla, then use chocolate to pipe on words, or vice versa.

These ideas are meant to be guidelines, to encourage you to try your own improvisations. Just plain old fruit by itself is a lovely and quick dessert too, so you never have to be without some sweetness in your life.

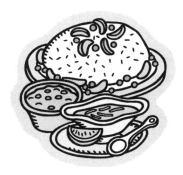

Healthy Dark Chocolate

🕐   **6 tablespoons melted organic coconut oil**
      1 tablespoon dark organic cocoa powder (preferably Fair-Trade)
      1 teaspoon organic vanilla
      ½ to 1 teaspoon Stevia or Lo Han, to taste
      1 tablespoon ground Salba, chia or shelled sunflower seeds
       (grind in coffee grinder dedicated to this purpose)
      1 tablespoon shredded coconut if desired (optional)
      Individual raisins or nuts, as desired.

1. Melt the coconut oil by setting its jar into a pan of simmering water.
2. Put cocoa, sweetener, and vanilla into a Pyrex glass measuring cup.
3. Pour melted coconut oil into it. If it is cold weather, you may need to set the measuring cup into the hot water to prevent the oil from solidifying.
4. Stir mixture until smooth.
5. Taste and adjust sweetener, if needed.
6. Stir in seeds, and, if using, shredded coconut.
7. Once well mixed, pour into your mold of choice. (Ice cube tray, soap making mold, silicon bakery mold, etc.)
8. Let set slightly, then add raisins or nuts gently so that they stay suspended.
9. Put molds into the refrigerator until firm—about 10-15 minutes.
10. Pop them out of molds and enjoy! Store uneaten chocolate in the fridge.

🕐 *Indicates something that needs to be done ahead of time*

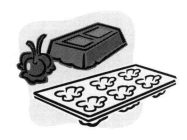

Chocolate Covered Strawberries

🕐   **6 tablespoons melted organic coconut oil**
     1 tablespoon dark organic cocoa powder (preferably Fair-Trade)
     1 teaspoon organic vanilla
     ½ to 1 teaspoon Stevia or Lo Han, to taste
     1 tablespoon ground Salba, chia, or raw sunflower seeds
     Strawberries, cherries, bananas or other fruit of your choice

1. Melt coconut oil by setting its jar into a pan of simmering water.
2. Put cocoa, sweetener, and vanilla into a Pyrex glass measuring cup.
3. Pour the melted coconut oil into it. If it is cold weather, you may need to set the measuring cup into the hot water to keep the oil from solidifying.
4. Stir mixture until smooth, and pour into a pint-sized jar.
5. Taste and adjust sweetener, if needed.
6. Hold strawberry or other fruit by its top and dip into the chocolate.
7. Take out and set on a plate. Enjoy when all are dipped!
8. Don't put these into the refrigerator or they will stick to the plate.

If it's summer, you can just set the jar of coconut oil out in the sun to melt.

🕐 *Indicates something that needs to be done ahead of time*

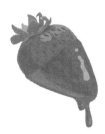

G.O.R.P. Bars

Good Old Raisins and Peanut Butter
(Makes 24 Squares)

1½ cups sweetened raw peanut butter (Valencia is a good one)
½ cup coconut oil
1 cup chopped almonds or pecans
1 cup unsweetened coconut (shredded)
1 cup raw sunflower seeds
1 cup raisins
2 teaspoons vanilla
2 tablespoons Salba or chia seeds

1. Heat the peanut butter, vanilla, and coconut oil in a 2-cup Pyrex measuring cup placed in simmering water, until melted and smooth.
2. In a bowl, mix together nuts, shredded coconut, sunflower seeds, Salba or chia seeds, and raisins.
3. Add melted mixture to the dry ingredients; mix until well combined.
4. Pour into a 9x13" casserole dish and press flat.
5. Cut into squares and enjoy.
6. Store in an airtight container.

To make a half recipe, use an 8x8" pan and cut all the ingredients in half.

Ideally, the nuts and seeds should be soaked overnight before making these, but I have to admit I don't usually do that.

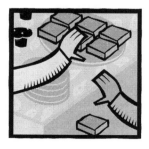

Coconut Walnut Date Rounds

Makes 24 rounds

🕐   **1½ cups walnuts (soaked overnight and drained)**
🕐   **1½ cups dates (soaked 1-2 hours)**
        ½ cup unsweetened cocoa powder
        1 teaspoon cinnamon
        ¼ cup unsweetened coconut milk
        Coconut flakes to roll rounds in

1. Put walnuts and dates into a food processor and process.
2. Add cocoa powder and cinnamon and process again.
3. Mix in the coconut milk until thoroughly blended.
4. Take out and form into 1-inch balls.
5. Roll in coconut flakes and eat (or freeze some for later).

🕐 *Indicates something that needs to be done ahead of time*

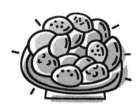

Desserts

Snow Balls

Makes approximately 2 dozen

🕐 **1 cup cashews (soaked overnight and drained)**
🕐 **6-10 dates, pitted; cover with water, soak 4 hours (reserve juice)**
½ cup finely blended coconut flakes (as opposed to shredded)
½ teaspoon vanilla
1 teaspoon cinnamon
Date juice from soaking

1. Blend nuts until finely chopped in a food processor or Vitamix blender.
2. Add coconut flakes, vanilla, dates (with their water), and cinnamon; blend.
3. Form dough into round balls about one inch in diameter.
4. Roll balls in extra coconut flakes to cover.
5. Refrigerate for two hours to set. Enjoy!

🕐 *Indicates something that needs to be done ahead of time*

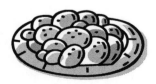

Fruit Roll-ups or Rounds

Very ripe fruit such as bananas, strawberries, blueberries, etc.

1. Take any fruit that is overripe and puree it in a blender.
2. Spread puree out on a Teflex sheet and put into dehydrator.
3. Dehydrate at 105°F for 6-8 hours.
4. Peel off the Teflex sheet halfway through and leave the roll-ups on the mesh sheet for the remainder of the time.
5. When done, add a filling if desired, and roll up.
6. Cut into 4-6" sections, and serve.

You can also drop the puree onto a Teflex sheet as small, round circles and dehydrate the same way. These can be little candies by themselves or you can add a filling of your choice, and fold in half.

If you don't have a dehydrator, you can put them in your oven on the lowest setting and leave the door open a bit. They won't be raw but they will firm up. Watch to see how long you should leave them in. Ovens vary greatly.

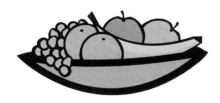

Pie Crust
Makes two pie crusts

🕐   **2 cups almonds (soaked overnight – they will expand)**

🕐   **1 cup soaked dates (barely cover dates and soak for an hour; reserve water)**

       1 teaspoon sea salt

       2 teaspoons vanilla

Note: Be sure to check the dates before putting them in the processor to make certain there are no pits. Even if you think you have pitted dates, there can sometimes be seeds left behind. This can tear up your food processor blades.

1. Blend all together (including water from dates) in the food processor until nuts are chopped well.
2. Divide mixture in half and make two pie crusts.
3. Press the mixture onto the pie plate until it is all covered.
4. Put in freezer, or dehydrate, or use as is.

🕐 *Indicates something that needs to be done ahead of time*

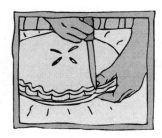

Macadamia Mango Pie
Serves 8

🕐 **1 cup macadamia nuts (soaked 8 hours and drained)**
4 mangos, peeled
¼ teaspoon Lo Han or Stevia (Lo Han would be better because it is a fruit extract and would add a fruity taste)
1 teaspoon vanilla
1 teaspoon sea salt
2 teaspoons cinnamon
1 lime, freshly juiced
2 teaspoons ground Salba or chia seeds (or more to thicken)
1 date nut pie crust (see recipe on page 214)

1. Place macadamia nuts, mango, sweetener, vanilla, salt, cinnamon, and lime juice in a food processor and process until smooth.
2. Add Salba or chia seeds and blend well.
3. Let mixture sit for 30 minutes to thicken. If needed, add more Salba.
4. Spoon into prepared date nut pie crust and serve. May be frozen.

If you prefer not to have a pie crust, this can be used as a pudding; any left-over filling that won't fit into the pie crust can be kept as pudding.

🕐 *Indicates something that needs to be done ahead of time*

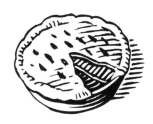

Blueberry Pie
Serves 8

Filling:

4 cups blueberries (five 4.4 ounce containers)
10 Medjool or Deglet dates
¼ teaspoon vanilla extract

1. Put 2 cups of blueberries (three 4.4 oz. containers) plus dates and vanilla into a food processor and blend until smooth.
2. Add the other cups (two 4.4 oz containers) of blueberries and mix.
3. Take mixture out and pour into the date nut piecrust (recipe below).
4. Let sit to thicken, as the natural pectin in the blueberries causes it to jell.

Pie Crust:

🕐 **1 cup almonds soaked 8 hours or overnight and drained**
🕐 **½ cup soaked dates (barely cover dates and soak for an hour; reserve water)**
½ teaspoon sea salt
1 teaspoon vanilla

1. Always check the dates for pits, even if purchased pitted.
2. Chop the soaked almonds in a food processor until coarsely ground.
3. Add the dates with their water, and process until chopped well.
4. Add the salt and vanilla, and blend well.
5. Take the crust mixture out and spread it over the bottom of a pie plate.

🕐 *Indicates something that needs to be done ahead of time*

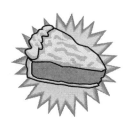

Peach Cobbler

Serves 8

6-8 peaches (depending on size), peeled and pits removed

🕐 5 pitted dates or more, to taste (soaked 1-2 hours)

½ teaspoon sea salt

2 teaspoons cinnamon

2 teaspoons Salba or chia seeds

1 crust mixture (see recipe below)

1. Place half of the peaches, dates (<u>without</u> their water), and salt in a Vitamix or food processor, and blend well.
2. Add Salba or chia seeds, blending well, and let sit for 15 minutes.
3. Chop the remaining peaches coarsely, and put them in a bowl.
4. Blend the peach mixture again, and add to the chopped peaches.
5. Pour into a glass pie or casserole dish.
6. Crumble the crust mixture (below) and stir into cobbler; serve.

Crust mixture

🕐 1 cup almonds (soaked 8 hours or overnight, and drained)

🕐 ½ cup soaked dates (barely cover dates and soak for an hour; reserve water)

Combine all ingredients, <u>including</u> water, in a food processor and mix coarsely.

🕐 *Indicates something that needs to be done ahead of time*

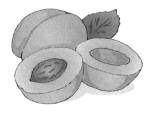

Desserts

Apple Pie
Serves 8

6 apples of your choice, either sweet (red or golden delicious) or tart (Granny Smith), cored but not peeled
1 teaspoon sea salt
2 teaspoons cinnamon
1 teaspoon vanilla
3 dates, pitted, soaked 1 hour and drained
Dash of Stevia or Lo Han if, desired
1 cup raisins
1 tablespoon chia seeds, ground in dedicated coffee grinder

1. Place 4 apples, salt, cinnamon, vanilla, and soaked dates in food processor.
2. Process until mixture is almost like applesauce.
3. Taste and add sweetener, if desired. Lo Han, a fruit extract, works best.
4. Chop other apples coarsely and add (reserving some to slice for garnish).
5. Add raisins—they will soak up the juice from the apples.
6. Stir in ground chia seeds, mixing well.
7. Let stand at room temperature for 30 minutes. Mixture will thicken.
8. Place mixture in crust (see recipe on page 214). Garnish with apple slices.
9. Serve alone, or with ice cream or yogurt.

Indicates something that needs to be done ahead of time

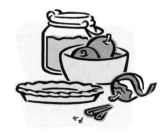

Raw Pumpkin Pie
Serves 8

2 cups chopped pumpkin (or butternut squash, or sweetpotatoes)
1 cup dates, soaked 1-2 hours
2 teaspoons cinnamon
1 teaspoon nutmeg
1 teaspoon coconut oil
Dash of vanilla
¼ cup raw milk (your choice), or water to help blend

Optional Topping (instead of whipped cream):

Raw yogurt, preferably home-made
Stevia or Lo Han, to taste
Dash of vanilla

1. Take cubes of pumpkin and mix in a Vitamix blender until pureed.
2. Add rest of ingredients and blend until smooth.
3. Pour into a prepared raw crust (see recipe page 214)
4. Refrigerate for 30 minutes before serving.
5. Top with yogurt topping if you can't get raw cream for whipping.

Note: Be sure to use "Pie" pumpkin, not jack-o-lantern pumpkin.

🕐 *Indicates something that needs to be done ahead of time*

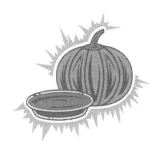

Desserts

Butterscotch Pudding

Serves 4

**1 cup dried apricots, soaked overnight in water
(make sure there's no sulfur dioxide—organic stores have them)
2 bananas, peeled
8 dates, soaked for 20 minutes (reserve water)
¼ cup coconut milk
¼ cup almond butter**

1. Combine all ingredients in a food processor or Vitamix and blend well.
2. Use as much of the soak water as needed for a pudding-like consistency.
3. Serve in pudding cups or ramekins.

This resembles the real thing, which you may remember as comfort food from your youth. Take a trip down memory lane with this healthy substitute.

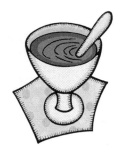

Salbioca Pudding
Serves 1

If you remember tapioca pudding from your childhood and long for it again, but don't want to spend hours waiting for it to cook, you're in luck! This recipe approximates it well without the HFCS and other junk of packages today.

This is the one time I recommend splurging on the more expensive Salba seeds, rather than using chia seeds. Not only are they nutritionally superior (see page 54 on Salba), but they more closely resemble the real thing.

Individual serving:

¾ cup raw milk of choice (cow, goat, almond, rice, coconut, etc.)
⅛ cup Salba seeds
Dash of vanilla
Stevia to taste

1. Put all ingredients into a jar with a lid.
2. Put lid on jar and shake to disburse all the seeds evenly.
3. Store in refrigerator overnight. The seeds will soak up the milk and thicken it just like tapioca.
4. Pour into a tall glass and enjoy, or just eat it out of the jar!

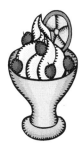

Banana Date Pudding
Serves 12

Crust:

⏰ **1 cup of almonds (soaked overnight and drained)**
⏰ **½ cup of dates, pitted (soaked 1-2 hours, reserve water)**
½ teaspoon salt
1 teaspoon vanilla

1. Place all in food processor, mix to crumbles. Add date soak water if needed.
2. Cover the bottom of a 9x9" square glass dish with half of the crust.

Pudding:

4 very ripe bananas
⏰ **4 dates pitted (soaked 2 hours, reserve water)**
1 teaspoon vanilla
½ teaspoon sea salt
Date juice as needed
Extra bananas to slice and layer (two or three depending on size)

1. Place bananas in Vitamix and blend until smooth.
2. Add dates, vanilla, and salt, and blend *(Note: may use unsoaked dates)*.
3. Add date juice, if needed, to make a creamy pudding.
4. Cut extra bananas into round slices and spread over crust.
5. Pour banana pudding over them, and sprinkle extra crust on top.
6. Put extra layer of banana slices, and more pudding, before crust if desired.

Shelf life: 2 days if you can keep it around that long.

⏰ *Indicates something that needs to be done ahead of time*

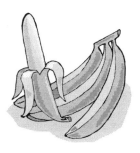

Alive Health Recipe Book

Lemon Cookies

Makes about 2 dozen cookies

4 eggs
1 cup Xylitol
1½ teaspoons lemon extract
¼ teaspoon sea salt
🕐 **½ cup butter, melted**
¾ cup sifted coconut flour

1. Pre-heat oven to 375°F.
2. Combine eggs, Xylitol, lemon extract, salt, and butter, and mix well.
3. Stir in coconut flour.
4. Let batter rest for 4-5 minutes to allow it to thicken slightly.
5. Drop batter in soup spoon-sized mounds 2" apart on greased cookie sheet (or use parchment paper for easier cleanup).
6. Bake at 375° for 15 minutes.

🕐 *Indicates something that needs to be done ahead of time*

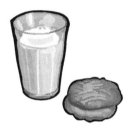

Zucchini Brownies

(Moms, here's how to add more veggies for the kids. They'll never notice.)

2 cups oatmeal flour, purchased or homemade
1½ cups Xylitol
1 teaspoon sea salt
1½ teaspoons baking soda
¼ cup organic cocoa powder, preferably Free Trade
½ cup coconut oil, melted
2 teaspoons vanilla
Splash of apple cider vinegar (to help it rise)
2 cups finely grated zucchini
½ cup nuts of your choice, optional

1. Preheat oven to 350°F.
2. Make flour if needed: grind 2½ cups of old-fashioned oats (not quick cooking) in a Vitamix or other blender until very fine, like flour.
3. Put flour into a bowl and add Xylitol, salt, baking soda, and cocoa powder.
4. Add coconut oil, vanilla, and apple cider vinegar; stir to mix.
5. Add zucchini, and mix well.
6. If using, fold in nuts.
7. Pour into a well greased 7x11" or 9x13" pan.
8. Bake at 350° for 35 minutes.
9. Cool completely before cutting.

Use parchment paper cut to fit your pan for easy clean-up afterwards.

Indicates something that needs to be done ahead of time

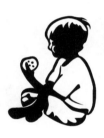

Raw Brownies
(Quick and easy to make; makes 1 dozen)

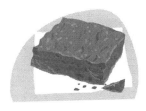 ¼ cup organic coconut oil, melted
¼ cup raw cocoa powder (preferably Fair Trade and Organic)
Dash of vanilla

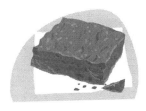 1 cup chopped walnuts, soaked 8 hours (*use unsoaked if really hungry*)

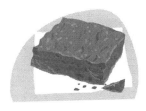 1 cup pitted dates (soaked 1-2 hours)

1. Melt coconut oil; put in pyrex measuring cup in pan of heated water.
2. Add cocoa powder and vanilla, and stir.
3. Put walnuts and pitted dates into a food processor and process slightly.
4. Add liquid ingredients and process until large ball forms, or until it stops turning properly.
5. Put mixture in a shallow pan and pat it down with your fingers to fit.
6. Cut to bite-sized pieces.
7. Put into the refrigerator for a few minutes to solidify, and then enjoy!

These don't keep for a long time so you'll have to make small batches and eat them fairly quickly. That is usually not a problem, since they're delicious!

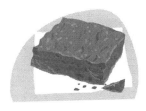 *Indicates something that needs to be done ahead of time*

Chocolate Pecan Cookies

Makes about 16 cookies

¼ cup butter or coconut oil
⅓ cup organic cocoa powder
3 eggs, preferably free-range
⅓ cup Xylitol
¼ teaspoon sea salt
¼ teaspoon organic vanilla
¼ cup sifted coconut flour
¼ cup chopped pecans

1. Preheat oven to 350°F.
2. In an enameled saucepan over low heat, melt butter, and stir in cocoa.
3. Remove from heat and let cool.
4. In a bowl combine eggs, Xylitol, sea salt, and vanilla, and stir into cocoa.
5. Sift coconut flour into batter, and whisk until smooth.
6. Fold in pecans.
7. Let the batter rest for about 5 minutes, allowing it to thicken slightly.
8. Drop batter by spoonfuls onto a cookie sheet covered with parchment paper (clean-up is easier and food doesn't touch Teflon this way).
9. Bake at 350° for 14 minutes.

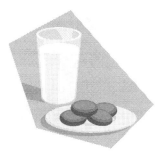

Cinnamon Roll Up

Makes about 10 servings

🕐
1 cup oats, ground to a flour in a Vitamix or food processor
1 cup golden flaxseed, ground to a flour
½ cup macadamia nuts, soaked 8 hours, dried, and ground
¼ cup extra virgin olive oil
¼ teaspoon Stevia or Lo Han in a little bit of water
Dash of sea salt
Water as needed to help form dough

1. Combine ground oat, flaxseed, and macadamia flour in a bowl.
2. Add olive oil, sweetener, and salt, and mix well, adding water as needed to form a firm ball of dough (will be a bit crumbly).
3. On flexible cutting board, spread dough thinly to form a rectangle.

🕐
½ cup dates, (soaked 1-2 hours—reserve water)
½ cup walnuts, soaked overnight
½ teaspoon sea salt
½ cup of soak water from dates
4 teaspoons cinnamon

1. Process all ingredients in Vitamix or food processor.
2. Put filling on top of dough, and roll up, keeping it together.
3. Cut dough into individual cinnamon swirl buns and serve, either for dessert or for breakfast.

🕐 *Indicates something that needs to be done ahead of time*

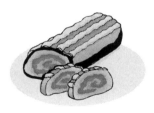

Desserts

Oatmeal Raisin Cookies

Makes about 25-26 cookies

2 cups oat flour, purchased or made in Vitamix or food processor

🕐 **1 cup cashews (soaked overnight)**

¼ teaspoon Stevia or Lo Han, to taste

2 teaspoons cinnamon

🕐 **1 cup raisins, soaked 1-2 hrs (barely cover with water and reserve)**

1. Put oat flour into a bowl.
2. After rinsing, grind the cup of soaked cashews and add to bowl.
3. Blend raisins, with their water, in a Vitamix or food processor.
4. Add sweetener and cinnamon to the raisins.
5. Pour raisin mixture into flour and blend. (May need to add more water.)
6. After mixing thoroughly, form into balls about 1" in diameter and flatten to quarter inch rounds.
7. You can eat these raw, or dehydrate them for 3-6 hours at 105°, or bake them in your oven at its lowest setting. They are really good!

Note: Can be frozen and baked later.

🕐 *Indicates something that needs to be done ahead of time*

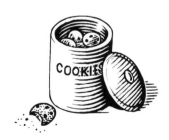

Raw Milk Ice Cream

Makes 4 half cup Servings

1 cup raw goat or cow milk
½ cup Xylitol
¼ cup (1 scoop) Dr. Mercola's Whey Protein (your choice flavor)
1 teaspoon vanilla
4 cups ice cubes

1. Mix all ingredients in order listed, except ice cubes, in a Vitamix blender.
2. Blend until smooth.
3. Add ice cubes and blend again, this time on high for 30-60 seconds.
4. When four mounds form, stop blender, pour into dishes, and serve.
5. Do not over mix or it will melt.

You may add any fruit of your choice, either on top, or mixed within.

Do not use any whey product other than Dr. Mercola's. All others have too many adverse ingredients. *(See "Proper Protein for Shakes" on page 38)* .

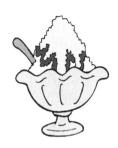

Desserts

Quick Coconut Vanilla Ice Cream

Sugar-free and Dairy-free Ice Cream
(Makes about 2 servings)

1 can (14 ounces) coconut milk
2 tablespoons Xylitol
Dash of sea salt
1 tablespoon vanilla

1. Combine coconut milk, Xylitol, and sea salt in a saucepan.
2. Heat at moderate to low temperature until ingredients are dissolved.
   Do not boil!
3. Take off heat and stir in vanilla.
4. If you have an ice cream maker, put mixture into refrigerator until chilled.
   Then follow directions given with your unit.

Otherwise, put mixture into an ice cube tray and freeze for two hours, until soft-serve consistency. Then put into a blender or Vitamix, and blend until consistency of a milkshake. Eat immediately or pour mixture into an airtight container and refreeze. Blending mixture and freezing it a second time crushes ice crystals that form during first freezing and gives the ice cream a smoother, creamier texture.

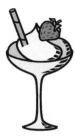

Zucchini Ice Cream

Serves 2

I kid you not, your kids will love it!

- 🕐 **1 cup frozen zucchini chunks or white pancake squash chunks**
- 🕐 **½ cup frozen banana chunks (or a small banana, frozen)**
- **⅛ teaspoon Stevia or Lo Han, to taste**

1. Put zucchini and banana chunks in a Vitamix or food processor.
2. Blend or process until creamy. You may need to use a bit of water if blades of Vitamix start to strain. Use tamper to get it all blended.
3. Add sweetener to taste.
4. Serve immediately so it doesn't melt.

If the ice cream starts to melt, put it back in the freezer for awhile. Stir it when you take it out, or blend again, if need be. If you leave the skin on the zucchini, it looks green—great for Halloween! To look more like vanilla ice cream, use white pancake squash instead.

This is a good way to use up extra zucchini when it's coming out your ears in August, and to get your kids to eat more vegetables. They'll never notice it.

🕐 *Indicates something that needs to be done ahead of time*

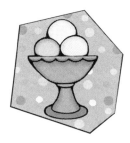

Chocolate Cake

½ cup butter
2 cups Xylitol
½ cup cocoa powder, preferably organic and Fair Trade
2 eggs
3 cups oat flour, purchased or homemade*
2 teaspoons aluminum-free baking powder
1 teaspoon salt
2 teaspoons vanilla
1½ cups raw milk
A splash of apple cider vinegar (to make it rise)

1. Preheat oven to 375°F.
2. Cream butter, sugar, and cocoa powder together.
3. Add eggs and mix well.
4. Gradually beat milk and vanilla into creamed mixture.
5. Mix flour, baking powder, and salt together in a separate bowl.
6. Beat dry ingredients into wet until smooth.
7. Pour into greased 9x13" pan, two 9" pans, or three 8" pans.
8. Bake at 375° for 35-40 minutes or until a toothpick comes out clean.
9. Cool, frost if desired, and serve. For vanilla cake, leave out the cocoa and add a teaspoon of lemon or almond extract, if desired.

*Make oat flour by grinding 3¾ cups old-fashioned oatmeal in a Vitamix.

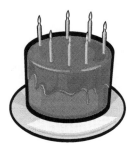

Vanilla Frosting

Makes 2½ cups

2 egg whites
1 cup Xylitol
¼ teaspoon cream of tartar
¼ cup water
1 teaspoon Vanilla

1. Combine egg whites, Xylitol, cream of tartar, and water in the top of a double boiler.
2. Beat at high speed for 1 minute.
3. Bring water in the bottom of double boiler to a rapid boil. Beat frosting for another 7 minutes or until peaks form when the beater is raised.
4. Transfer frosting to a large bowl.
5. Add vanilla extract and beat until thoroughly mixed.

Generously fills and frosts two 8" or 9" layers, or a 9x13" sheet cake.

If desired, cherry flavoring may be substituted for the vanilla extract.

Note: You can use the two egg yolks that are left over to make Mayonnaise, or Quick Hollandaise Sauce.

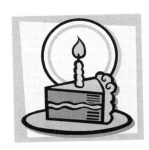

Chocolate Frosting
Sugar-free and Dairy-free
(Makes 2 cups)

🕐 **6 tablespoons coconut oil, melted**
2 cups Xylitol, sifted
½ cup unsweetened organic cocoa powder, sifted
8 tablespoons coconut milk (or cow's milk if not going dairy-free)
1 teaspoon vanilla

1. With electric mixer, beat melted coconut oil until creamy.
2. Sift Xylitol and cocoa powder together, in a separate bowl.
3. Gradually add dry ingredients to coconut oil, alternately with milk, until dry ingredients are dissolved. If too thick, heat gently.
4. Stir in vanilla.
5. Let sit until it has cooled and thickened to a spreadable consistency.
6. Spread frosting on top of cake or cupcakes. (Put frosting into a baggie and snip the corner to pipe words or draw, if desired.)

Note: If you use unsweetened, organic coconut milk in a carton, it will last 7 to 10 days. If using organic canned, it will only last 4 days.

🕐 *Indicates something that needs to be done ahead of time*

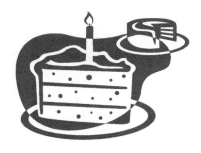

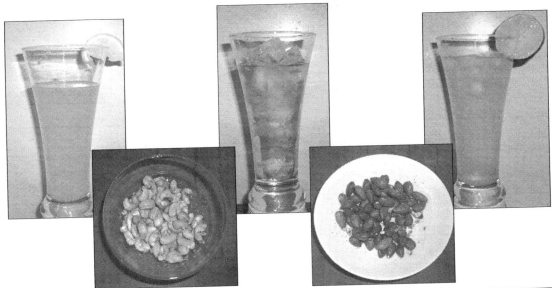

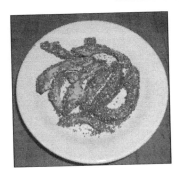

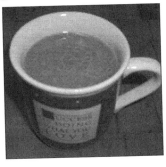

Beverages
And Snacks

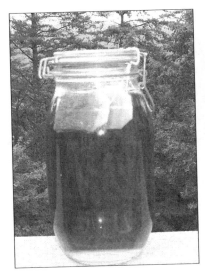

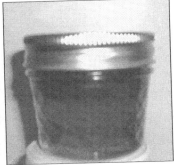

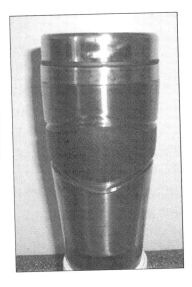

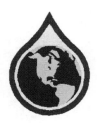

Beverages and Snacks

This section has beverages and snacks that, while very tasty, still keep you on your healthy eating pathway. Of course, the desserts or muffins can be eaten as a snack. Raw cheese is great, as well (my personal favorite). But these recipes offer you a few new snack choices.

Proper Hydration

If you really want to be healthy, the best thing you can do for yourself is to stop drinking sodas and commercially prepared drinks (Starbucks, fruit juices, etc.). Not only are they loaded with calories and sweetened with junk (either high fructose corn syrup, sugar, or artificial sweeteners—see pages 17-20), the body does not recognize them as food.

The body says, "Thanks for the hydration, now where's the real deal?" This is true even of fruit juices. If you are going to have fruit, which is good, eat the whole thing, not just the juice. That way you get the beneficial fiber along with it, not just empty calories (from the body's perspective).

The ideal thing would be to replace those drinks with fresh, pure spring water. Since I know that's not likely to happen (I *am* a realist), you may drink tea that you make yourself. Green tea is an excellent choice and has many good-for-you properties. You can make it by the cup, and pour the hot tea into a traveling mug. Or, you might want to make it by the half-gallon, as sun tea. See the recipe coming up for how to do that.

Take some tea along with you to work. Use a bottle, preferably glass. If that isn't practical, use a stainless steel container (something similar to an old-fashioned thermos). Tea loses its potency after 24 hours so try to drink it in one day, if possible. Herbal, white, or black tea also works well, and gives you an almost endless variety of choices. You'll save yourself a lot of money over vending machines, too.

Now the reality is, you want something sweet, right? Don't we all! Please DO NOT use any of the artificial sweeteners on the market—the pink, blue or yellow packets. They are very unsafe, but I won't go into that here. Just look at the pages cited above.

There is an alternative that is awesome and you will find it in the supplement section of your local health food store. It is called Stevia and is a naturally occurring herb native to South America that has been used since pre-Columbian times. It comes in liquid and powder form, as well as in single serving packets.

Natural Sweeteners Now Available

The FDA has finally approved Stevia to be used as a sweetener, and there are many brands now in the sweetener section. Truvia® and Pure Via™ are two of them, but they have fillers in them to make a "normal" looking packet of sweetener. The law does not require them to list what those fillers are, so buyer beware. Most of the time it is some kind of sugar, like dextrose. You can still find the Stevia herb by itself in some places.

I personally love Now® brand Stevia Extract. It won't break down in heat so you can cook with it, and it makes wonderful baked goods. Stevia is 200-300 times sweeter than sugar, depending on the blend, so a little bit goes a very long way. If you use too much, it will have a bitter taste.

The Stevia Extract has a tiny spoon in it that is about the equivalent of a teaspoonful of sugar. So start out with a small amount and add more, to your taste, if needed. Stevia will not impact your blood sugar, so it is safe for diabetics. Some brands do have a bit of an anise after-taste to them. Experiment with different brands until you find one that you like.

You can also use an extract called Luo Han Guo, or Lo Han for short. It is from a fruit found in the mountainous regions of China, and therefore has a fruity taste to it. In my opinion, it is the best sweetener to use in teas or other drinks. Please see Chapter Three, page 55, for more in-depth information on both Stevia and Lo Han. Making a change is really important for your future good health.

Making a Simple Syrup

You can also make up a Simple Syrup, once you find the type if sweetener that you like best. It can be used to sweeten large batches of tea or any kind of drink. Several of the recipes include instructions for making the Simple Syrup.

Stevia Tea

4 tea bags of your choice (herbal, green, Tulsi, etc.)
Water
Simple Syrup

1. Put tea bags in a half-gallon container filled with cold water.
2. Place it in the sun for three to four hours; no more.
3. Bring it in and sweeten with the sweetener of your choice while it is still warm, or with Simple Syrup if it is cold.

Make the tea stronger and sweeter than normal if you are going to be putting it over ice in hot weather, because that will dilute it.

A deck or patio works fine for making sun tea, and is successful even in cold weather. If you don't have time to set it in the sun, you can put it in your refrigerator overnight.

Simple Syrup:

Take ½ teaspoon of Stevia or Lo Han and put it in ½ cup boiling water. Stir until it all dissolves. You can use this to sweeten cold or warm tea. If you have excess, store in a small jar in the refrigerator for 1-2 weeks.

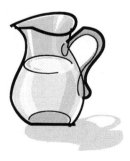

Lemonade

1 cup water
Juice from ½ of a fresh lemon
Simple Syrup

1. Add the lemon juice to a glass of cold, filtered or spring water.
2. Sweeten to taste with Simple Syrup.
3. If adding ice, make it sweeter because it will be diluted.

Simple Syrup:

Take ½ teaspoon of Stevia or Lo Han and put it in ½ cup boiling water. Stir until it all dissolves. You can use this to sweeten cold or warm tea, also. If you have excess, store in a small jar in the refrigerator for 1-2 weeks.

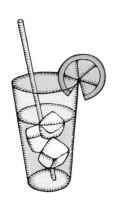

Limeade

1 cup water
Juice from ½ of a fresh lime
Simple Syrup

1. Add the lime juice to a glass of cold, filtered or spring water.
2. Sweeten to taste with Simple Syrup.
3. If adding ice, make it sweeter because it will be diluted.

Simple Syrup:

Take ½ teaspoon of Stevia or Lo Han and put it in ½ cup boiling water. Stir until it all dissolves. You can use this to sweeten cold or warm tea, also. If you have excess, store in a small jar in the refrigerator for 1-2 weeks.

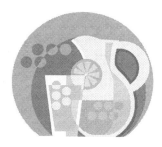

Hot Chocolate

1 mug of raw milk (cow, goat, almond, rice or coconut)
1 teaspoon organic, unsweetened cocoa powder (pref. Fair Trade)
¼ teaspoon Stevia or Lo Han
1 teaspoon coconut oil, or more, to taste

1. Heat milk in saucepan over low heat until just hot enough to drink. Test using a clean knuckle—when it is comfortable to your hand, it's done.
2. Add the cocoa powder and stir until it dissolves completely.
3. Add the sweetener and again, stir until it dissolves. Use a lot of sweetener, relatively speaking, to counteract the bitterness of the plain cocoa powder.
4. Add the coconut oil, to your taste. This adds a heavenly smoothness to the drink and you can add up to a tablespoon or more if you like.
5. Stir until smooth, find a nice fireplace and curl up beside it with your drink.

Coconut milk is now sold in cartons like regular milk, and it's organic. Be sure to get the original, unsweetened kind. Add your own healthy, good-for-you sweetener to your taste. This will last 7-10 days after opening so it gives you plenty of time to make lots of recipes with it.

Note: You can always add coconut oil to any hot teas that you make, too.

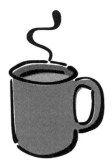

Cheesy Cashew Snack

🕐 **½ cup cashews, soaked overnight**
Olive oil or grapeseed oil to coat lightly
2 teaspoons of nutritional yeast, to taste
Pinch of sea salt

1. Drain the cashews, dry them and put them in a small bowl.
2. Drizzle with olive or grapeseed oil and mix to cover the nuts.
3. Add nutritional yeast and salt to your taste.
4. Enjoy them out of the bowl, or put them in a baggie if you're heading out.

Nutritional yeast can be found at most organic markets. (Do not use the red and yellow packets of bread yeast.) Optimally, it would be best to get raw cashews, but I know this is difficult. If you can only get roasted, salted nuts, don't bother soaking them since it won't help. Usually these are roasted in peanut or safflower oil so there is no danger of GMOs.

If using roasted nuts, omit the salt from above and only use the oil and nutritional yeast. These really taste cheesy, just like the unhealthy cheese puff-type snacks, and they will fill you up with goodness. Make some to keep on hand around the house.

🕐 *Indicates something that needs to be done ahead of time*

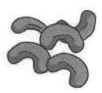

Cinnamon Almond Snack

🕐 ½ cup almonds (soaked overnight)
¼ teaspoon cinnamon
Dash of Stevia or Lo Han, to taste

1. Dry the soaked almonds on a paper towel to get most of the moisture off.
2. Sprinkle on cinnamon and sweetener, and mix together thoroughly.
3. Put these in a baggie if you're on the run, or eat them at home as desired.

Now who said you couldn't have healthy snacks? If you don't have time to soak the nuts overnight, just rinse them carefully a few times to get dirt off and follow the above. It won't be the end of the world.

🕐 *Indicates something that needs to be done ahead of time*

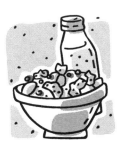

"Fried" Avocado Fritters

Makes 8-16

One ripe avocado
¼ cup chia or Salba seeds
Pinch of sea salt
Pinch of pepper
Pinch of cumin

1. Combine all but the avocado in a small bowl. This is your batter.
2. Slice a ripe avocado in half and remove the pit.
3. Cut each half into thin vertical slices, keeping intact, and remove peel.
4. Coat both sides of the avocado slices in the batter.
5. Put the slices on a mesh dehydrator tray with a Teflex sheet on the row below to catch any batter that falls. You can also put them on a cookie sheet lined with parchment paper and place in oven on its lowest setting. Do not attempt to turn the slices while baking.
6. Dehydrate until semi-crispy, about two to four hours or so.
7. Enjoy the crunch!

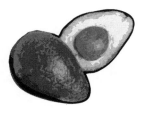

INDEX

Made in the USA
Charleston, SC
07 June 2012